THE GREAT FOAM ROLLER HANDBOOK

WRITTEN BY
Andre Noel Potvin

EDITED BY

CLINICAL EXERCISE & GENERAL FITNESS
Andre Noel Potvin
MSC, CSCS, CES

GENERAL EDITOR
Michael Jespersen

COPY EDITOR/WRITER
Aaron Driver

Second Printing
(December 2007)

Consult your physician before starting any exercise program. This is of particular importance if you are over 35 and have been inactive for a period of time. The author and publisher disclaim any liability from loss, injury, or damage, personal or otherwise, resulting from the procedures in this book.

We would like to thank Sissel for supplying the foam rollers for this handbook.

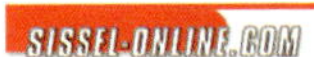

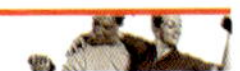

Published 2006
Productive Fitness Products Inc.
2289-135A St.
Surrey, B.C. V4A 9V2

Productive Fitness Products Inc.
1645 Jill's Court, Ste. 102
Bellingham, WA 98226

or e-mail
info@productivefitness.com

Visit our Website: www.productivefitness.com

Potvin, André Noël, 1961-
The great foam roller handbook / written by André Noël Potvin ; edited by André Noël Potvin ; general editor: Michael Jespersen; copy editor: Aaron Driver.

ISBN 0-9731262-6-4
1. Physical fitness--Handbooks, manuals, etc. I. Jespersen, Michael, 1962- II. Title. III. Title: Foam roller handbook.
RA781.P68 2006 613.7'1 C2006-905784-2

TABLE OF CONTENTS

Exercises

INTRODUCTION

Foam rollers are remarkably simple to use yet are almost infinite in their range of application. Because they are lightweight and economical, you can exercise almost anywhere in any position. Whether standing, sitting, kneeling, or even lying in bed, you can use foam rollers to build strength and flexibility. And what's more, they are fun to use.

Foam rollers are cylindrical in shape, which means they challenge the body on more than one plane of movement (up, down, sideways, forward and back). These functional challenges enhance your balance reactions and strengthen the critical stabilizing, core muscles often overlooked in traditional exercise.

But in addition to leading edge functional exercises, foam rollers also serve as an ingenious tool for myofascial release. Myofascial release is a highly effective therapy that has been used for more than a century to heal chronic pain and injuries, and to improve flexibility, circulation, poor posture and relaxation. However, until recently it has required the time and expense of a professional physical therapist. Thanks to exciting new techniques with the foam roller, this is no longer the case.

Foam roller techniques can release the pain-causing adhesions between the fascia and other tissues in the body. Fascia is the dense web of connective tissue that permeates our body, covering and connecting our muscles, organs and bones. Whether your injuries are nagging or debilitating, myofascial techniques will aid the healing process – it is like having your own private masseuse and physical therapist.

By exercising and massaging with the foam roller, you will generate greater body awareness, you will re-educate and strengthen your muscles, and you will improve your endurance. You will also notice increased relaxation and improved circulation. And because they are quick and easy to use – unlike so many modern exercise programs – foam rollers are the perfect tool for the busy lifestyle.

WHAT YOU'LL NEED

Foam rollers

Rollers come in a variety of sizes and shapes.They are made from a dense foam, which allows them to retain their shape, even under heavy weight. The large cylindrical shaped rollers and the half rollers come in varying lengths. The set below can be made with two full-length round rollers and two full-length half rollers.

Just cut the rollers to size with a bread knife.

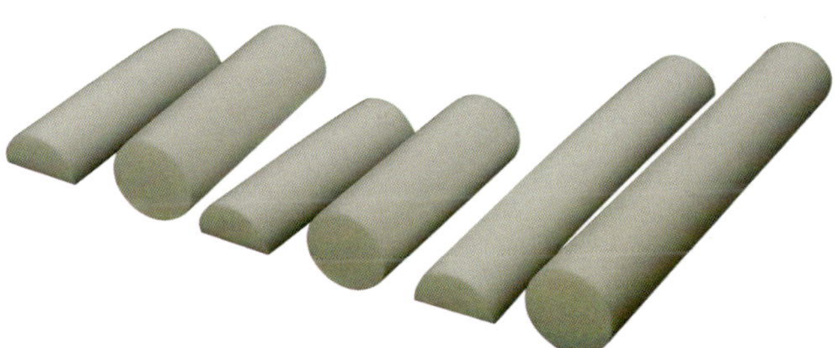

Inflatable rollers

Made from a sturdy material, an inflatable roller is a good option when travelling. However, these rollers are not designed to be stood on so exercises are limited.

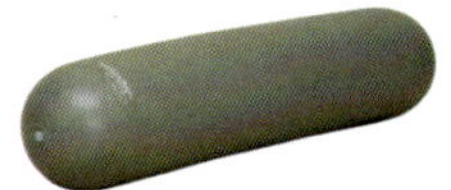

FitBall® Roller

Broomstick, Ball, Stretch Tubing, Door Attachment and Dumbbells

Other than the foam rollers, a few pieces of equipment will be necessary to perform all the exercises in this book. Most of these products can be purchased from your local fitness equipment store or online retailer, except the broomstick which can be purchased at your local hardware store.

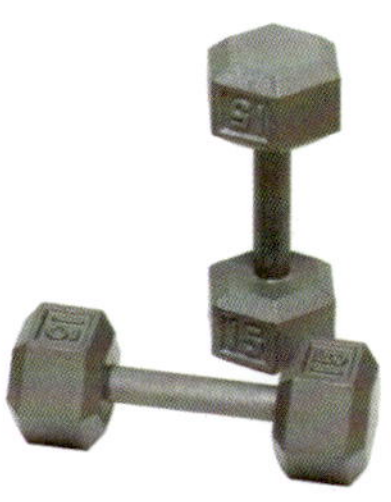

Dumbbells

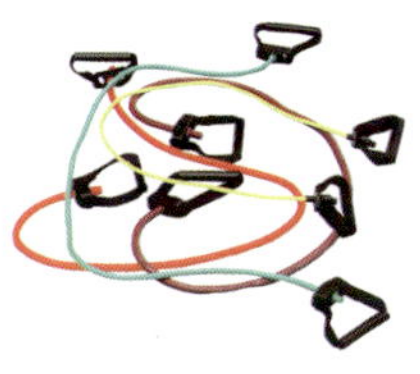

Stretch Tubing

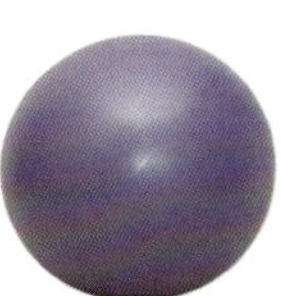

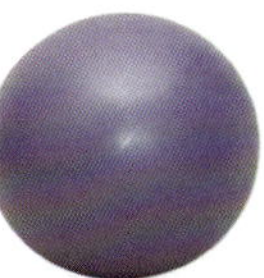

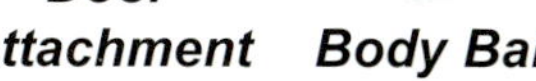

Door Attachment *Body Ball*

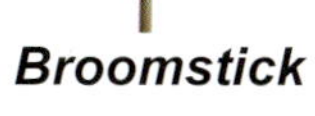

Broomstick

General Exercise GUIDELINES

- ✓ **Safely maximize your results:** For the first week or two of learning a new exercise, hold the "challenging position" for 5 seconds. This allows your body time to coordinate and develop your muscles safely and effectively, which will give better results over time. Increase the length of the hold time to 30 seconds before incorporating additional moves or increasing the speed of movement.
- ✓ **Always warm up before you start a workout:** Try to do a total-body warm-up before you start training. A good total-body warm-up is a light jogging motion for the lower body and modified push-ups for the upper body. It is especially important to warm up the specific muscle groups you are going to be exercising.
- ✓ **Use proper posture:** Maintaining proper posture will greatly reduce chances of injury and maximize your results. When standing, always keep your feet shoulder-width apart, unless otherwise instructed. Do not lock your knees: it puts an unnecessary strain on them. Keep your back flat and straight, making sure not to twist or arch it in order to complete an exercise.
- ✓ **Use proper exercise form:** Focus on the proper motion of the exercise, while concentrating on the specific muscles being used. Do not sacrifice proper form to perform more repetitions. Keeping proper form also means moving in a smooth fluid motion. Know when your muscles are too tired to keep going.
- ✓ **Breathe properly:** Never hold your breath during any part of an exercise. Holding your breath may cause severe intra-thoracic pressure and raise blood pressure, leading to dizziness, blackout, or worse. The rule of thumb is to exhale slowly on exertion and inhale on the return part of the exercise.
- ✓ **Stop training if you feel pain:** If you feel pain during a specific exercise, stop immediately. Any continuation may aggravate an existing injury. Decrease the amount of resistance you are using. Talk to a recognized health professional.
- ✓ **Use the Safe Exercise Flow Chart:** After each exercise go through the flow chart steps on the next page.

Safe Exercise FLOW CHART

(Soreness Test)

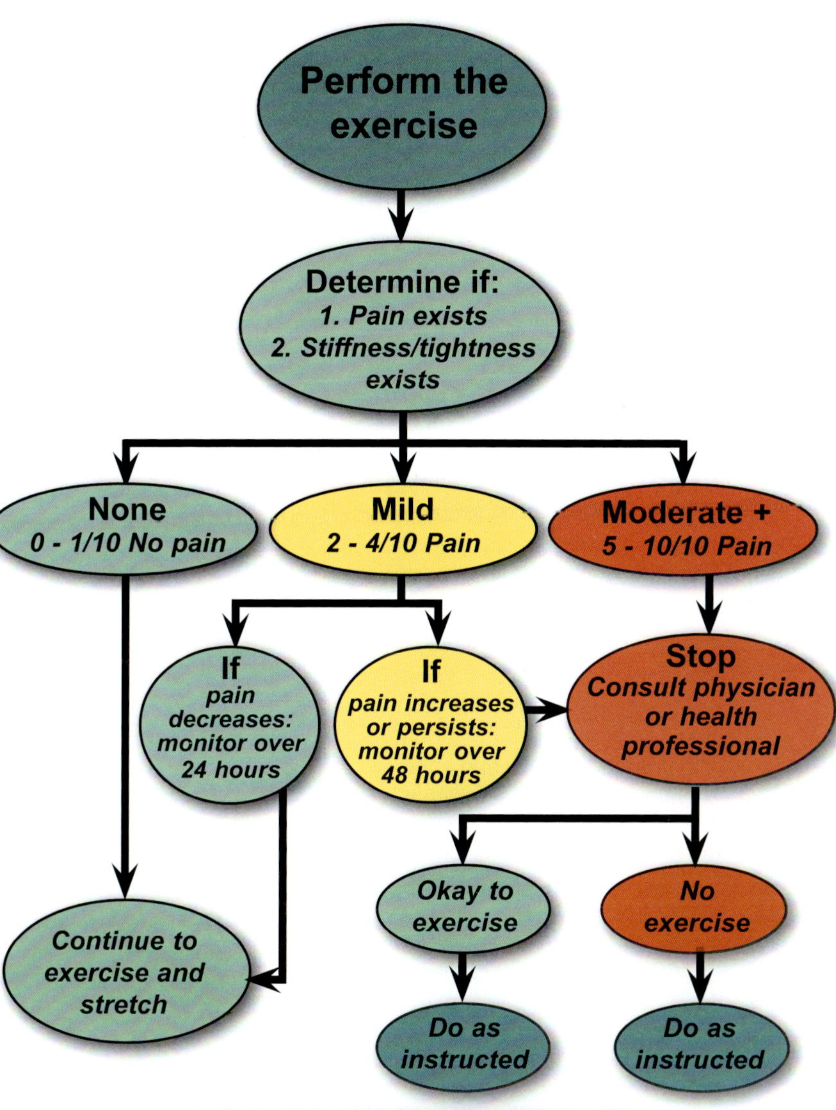

Pain Reference Scale

10 = Extreme pain
5 = Affects normal movement
3 = Does not affect normal movement
0 = No pain

Proper Posture and
THE GIRDLE GRIP

Slouch, then breathe in

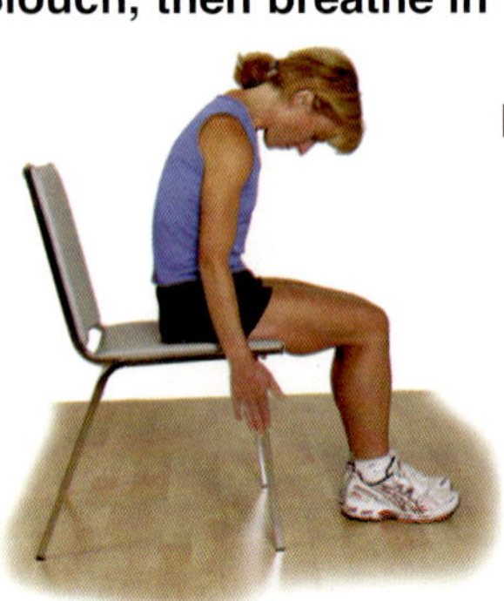

Breathe out and sit tall

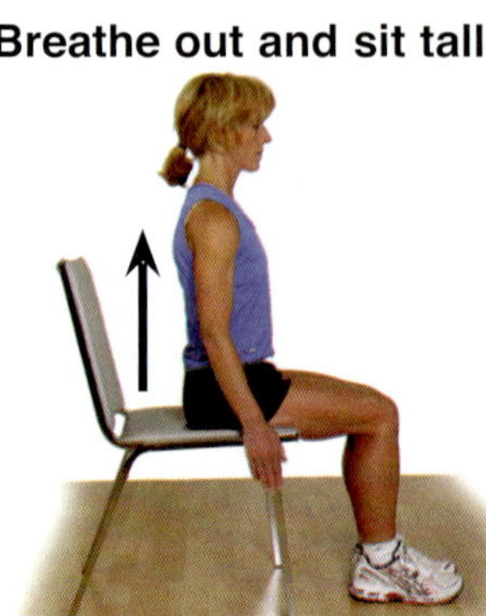

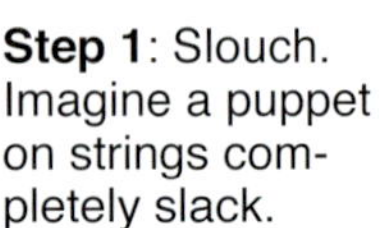

Step 1: Slouch. Imagine a puppet on strings completely slack.

Step 2: Breathe in while slouched.

Step 3: Breathe out through pursed lips while moving to a tall position. Imagine a puppet on strings being pulled tight.

Step 4: Continue exhaling and becoming taller. You should feel a contraction in your abdominals.

Step 5: Lock the contraction (this is the "Girdle Grip") and CONTINUE breathing.

Step 6: Try to maintain the Girdle Grip for one minute.

Benefits:

1. Establishes correct postural alignment. In this position your body has the least amount of stress from the effects of gravity.

2. Protects your lower back and spine when performing day to day activities, or even when performing occasional strenuous activity.

Tips: Practice this process often, when standing, sitting and walking.

Purpose: By training your muscles to perform the Girdle Grip on command you will protect your body, particularly your spine and lower back, from common injury.

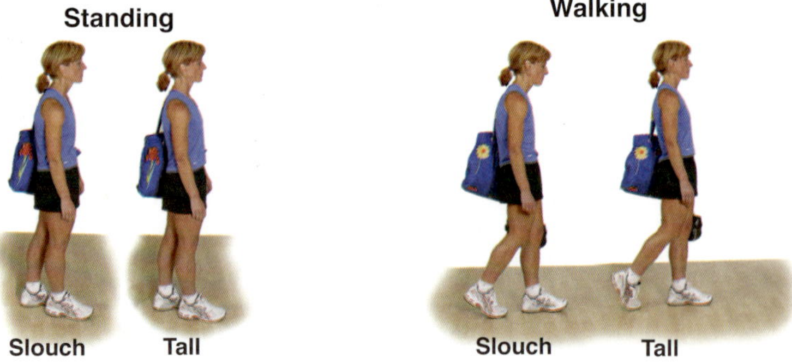

The Broomstick

One of the best ways to verify correct postural alignment is to hold a broomstick against your spine. The first time you try this, you might need someone to help you hold the stick and check your alignment. The stick is only used as a teaching or visualization aid. Once you understand its purpose, you only need to "think" of the stick when performing these activities.

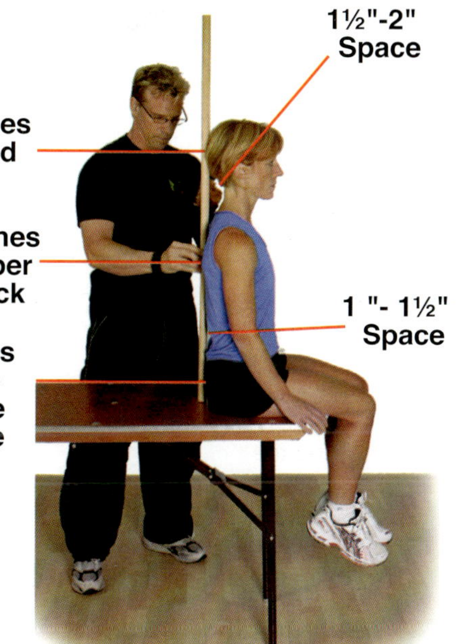

Regardless of whether you are sitting, standing, kneeling or on hands and knees, you should strive to achieve correct postural alignment. Maintain approximately 1½ to 2 inches of space between the stick and your cervical spine (back of neck), and 1 to 1½ inches at your lumbar spine (lower back). Your body should touch the broomstick in three places: the head, the upper back and the base of the spine (sacrum).

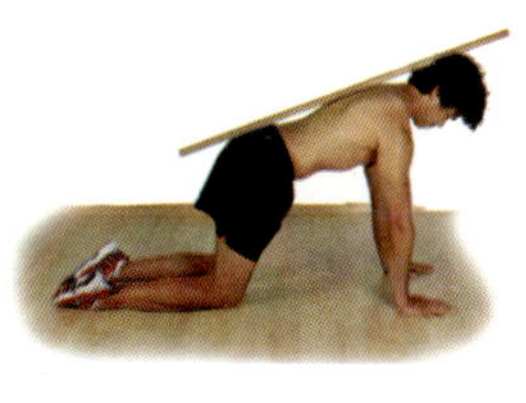

Note: Keep your chin parallel with the ground and keep your head neutral (not tilted up).

The broomstick can also be used to check the straightness of your body when performing other exercises.

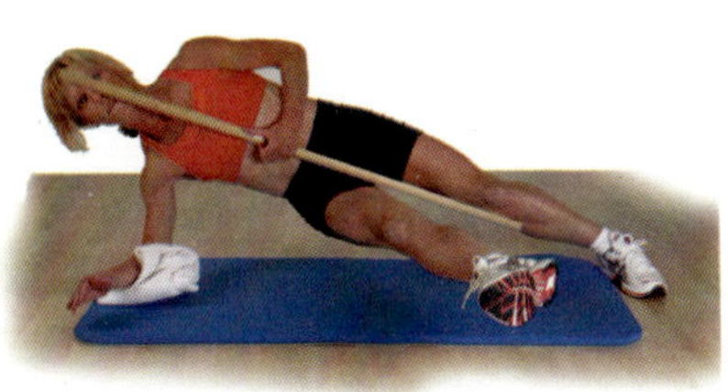

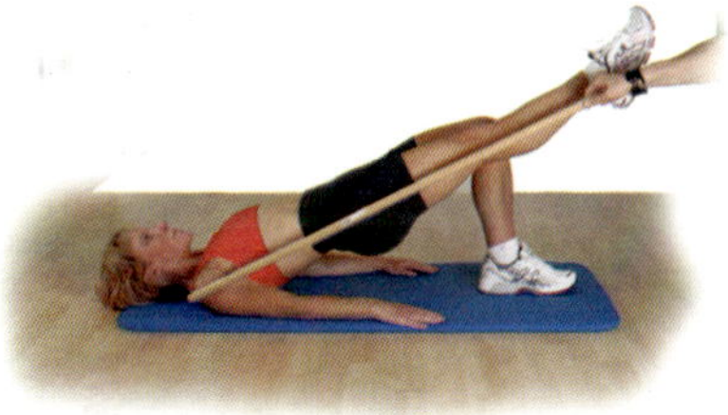

MUSCLE DIAGRAMS

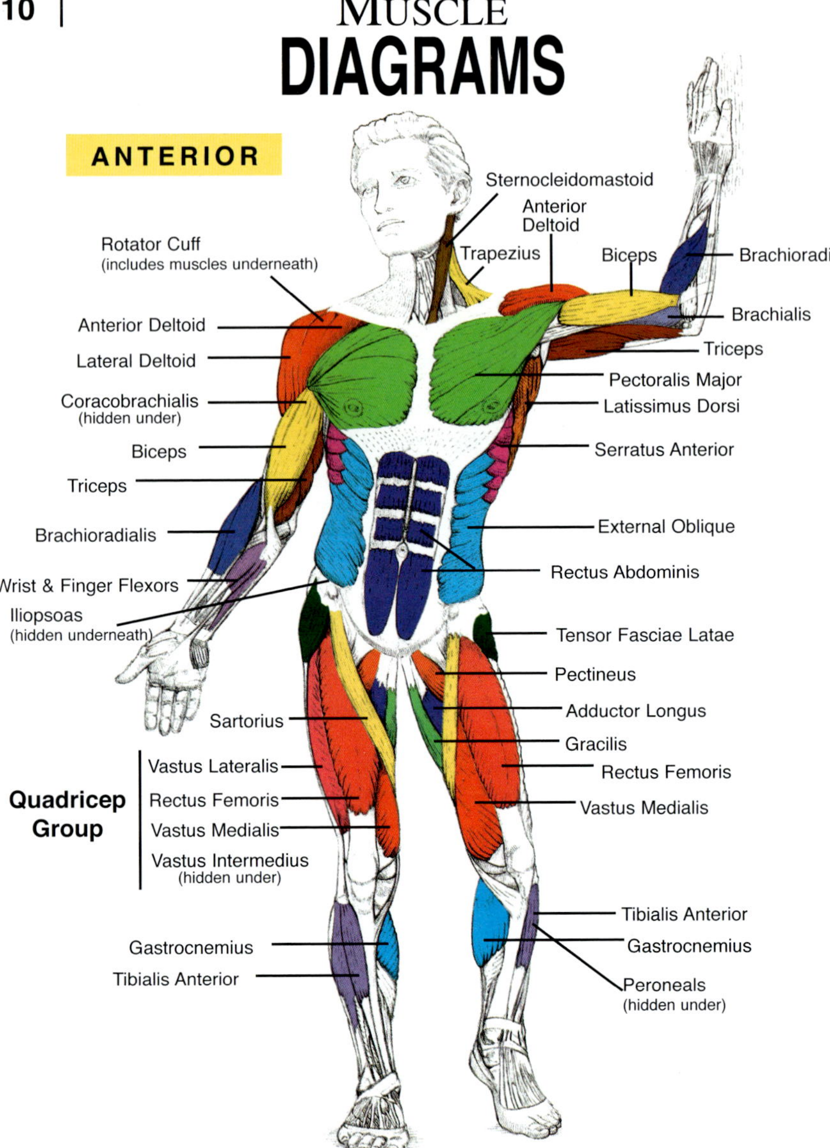

Neck Extensors	upper trapezius, illiocotalis cervicis, longissimus cervicis, spinalis cervicis. **Deep Extensors**: semispinalis cervicis, spinalis cervicis
Neck Retractors	longus colli, longus capitus
Scapular Depressors	latissimus dorsi, low trapezius
Scapular Retractors	rhomboids, mid-low trapezius
Shoulder Stabilizers	pectoralis major, deltoid, triceps (long head), latissimus dorsi, teres major, rotator cuff
Core (outer unit)	rectus abdominus, erector spinae, internal and external obliques
Core (inner unit)	pelvic floor muscles, diaphragm, multifidui, levator ani, transversus abdominus

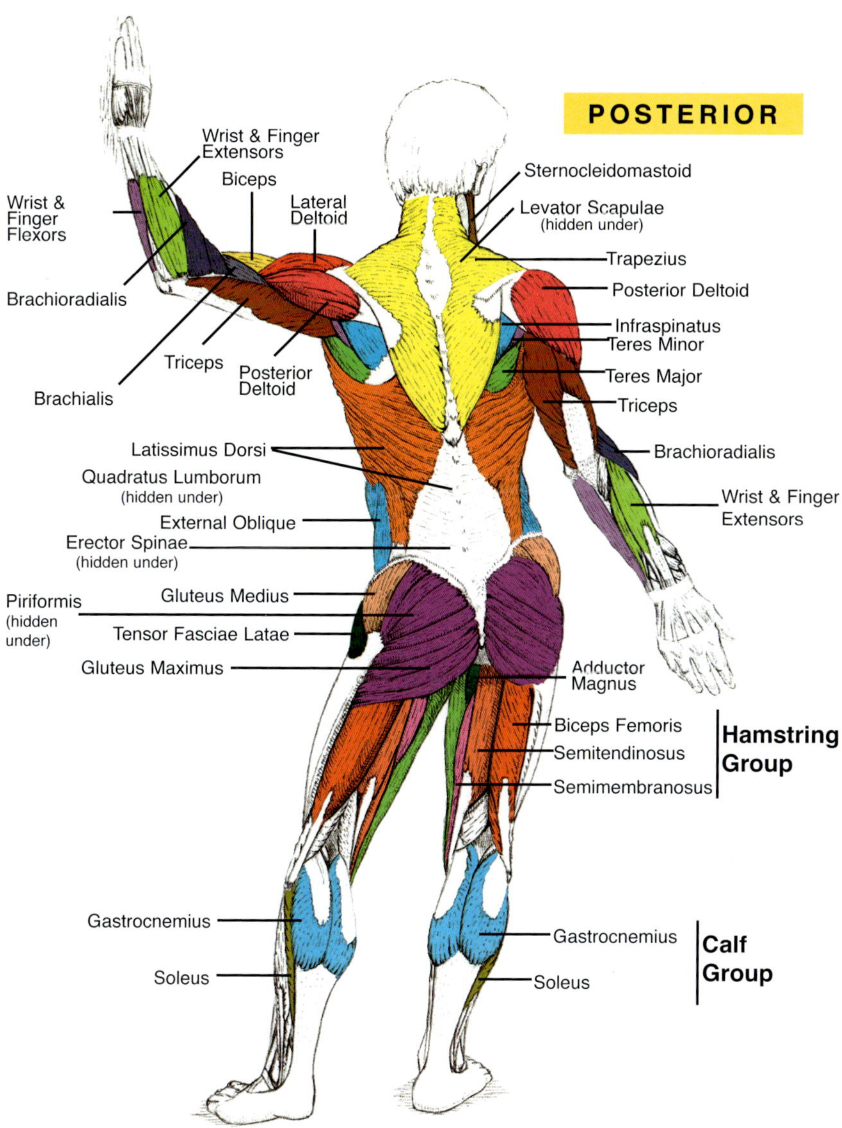

Pelvis Stabilizers	rectus abdominus, obliques, quadratus lumborum, latissimus dorsi
Spinal Rotators	obliques, erector spinae (unilaterally), rectus abdominus (unilaterally), deep spinal rotators
Hip Stabilizers	hip flexors, hip abductors, hip extensors, hip rotators
Hip Flexors	iliopsoas, sartorius, rectus femoris, tensor facia latae
Hip Adductors	adductor brevis, longus and magnus, gracilis, pectineus
Hip Extensors	gluteus maximus, hamstrings
Hip Abductors	gluteus medius and minimus, tensor fasciae latae, piriformis
Ankle Stabilizers	gastrocnemius, soleus, tibialis posterior, tibialis anterior, peroneals, extensor digitorum longus, brevis

STRETCHING

Why Stretch?

Regular stretching helps maintain and improve flexibility. The definition of flexibility is a joint's ability to move through a normal range of motion (ROM). Because each joint has its own degree of flexibility, it's possible to be very flexible in one joint and stiff in another. The primary limitation in joint ROM is the tough connective tissue running through the muscle belly. Other factors include:

- Age
- Genetics
- Previous activity (or lack of it)
- Joint structure (injury or no injury)
- Gender (women are generally more flexible than men)
- Body temperature (slightly warmer than normal increases flexibility)
- Opposing muscle tightness putting joints under stress.

By lengthening muscle and connective tissue, stretching reduces tension around a specific joint and allows it to move more freely. Other benefits of stretching include:

- Reduced joint stress due to muscular imbalances
- Reduced chronic soft-tissue pain (such as neck, back and knees)
- Increased relaxation
- Enhanced well-being

When stretching, keep the following points in mind:

- Stretch to a mild intensity (30% to 40% of maximum). The stretch should feel like a comfortable pull (no pain).
- Hold stretches for 30 to 60 seconds, until the muscle relaxes. When you begin a stretch, your muscles will feel tight. This feeling subsides as the muscle relaxes and then elongates.
- To enhance results, stretch when your muscles are warm, ideally after physical activity like resistance training or aerobics. Avoid stretching cold muscles.
- Pay extra attention to your tightest joints. Flexibility is joint-specific.
- Proper body alignment is critical. Carefully study and follow the stretch positions and explanations in this book.
- Breathe deeply as you stretch; this enhances relaxation by stimulating the Para Sympathetic Nervous System.

1 Head Tilts

(Stretches: scalenes, upper trapezius)

- Sit on a half roller placed from back to front, on your seat. Your feet should be spaced comfortably apart and flat on the floor. Tilt your head to the left and lower your right shoulder.
- Hold for 30 to 60 seconds; repeat 2 to 3 times. Switch sides.

Modification:

1. To gently intensify the stretch, place your right hand on the left side of head. Switch sides.

Caution: Be very gentle when intensifying this stretch.

2. Turn your head to look at your armpit while your head is tilted (picture shows head tilted to right).

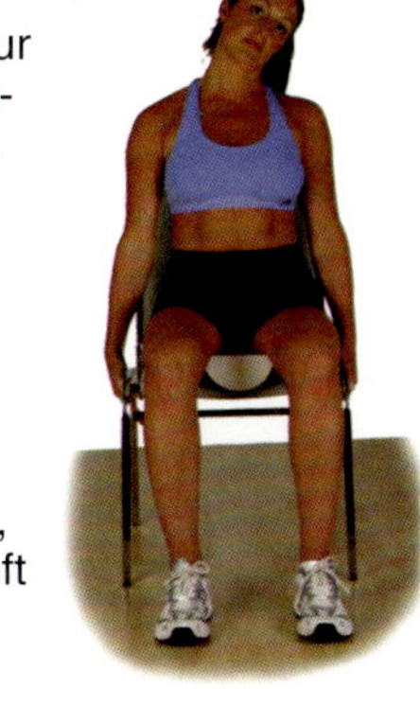

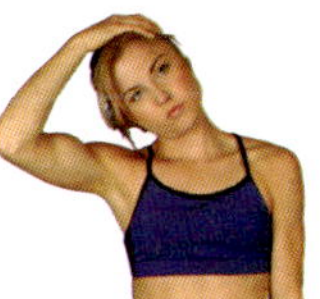

Hand on head

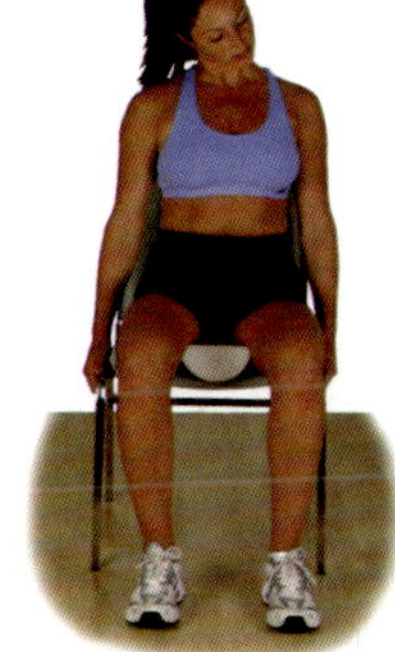

Head turn

2 Head Turns

(Stretches: neck rotators)

- Lie on a half roller (flat side down) so its lengthwise along your middle back and is supporting your head.
- Your feet should be spaced comfortably apart and flat on the floor.
- Place your left index and middle fingers on the right side of your jaw. Slowly turn your head to the left until you feel a comfortable stretch.
- Hold for 30 to 60 seconds and repeat 2 to 3 times. Switch sides.

Caution: Be very gentle when intensifying this stretch.

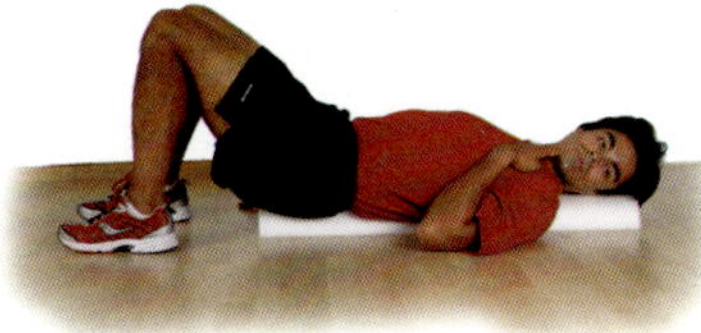

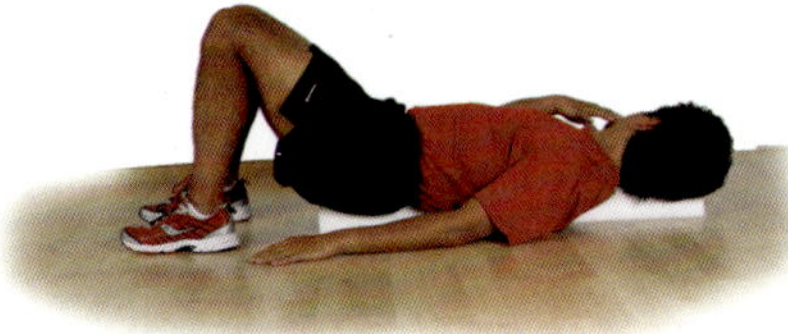

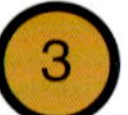

Hug Yourself

(Stretches: rhomboids, middle and lower trapezius)

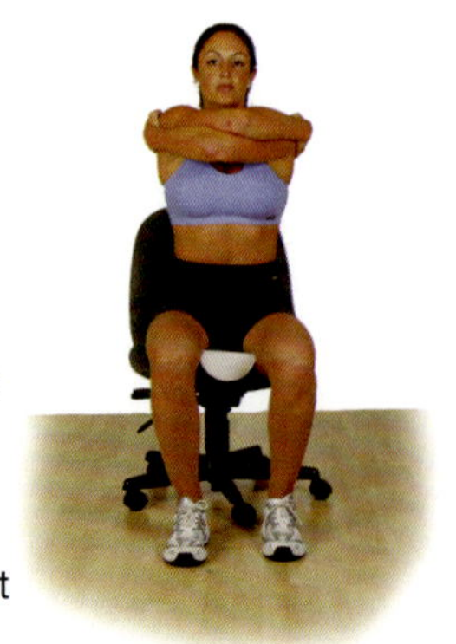

- Sit on a half roller placed from the back to the front of your seat. Your feet should be hip-width apart on the floor.
- Hug yourself: reach each hand to grab the opposite shoulder.
- Raise your elbows so they are almost parallel to the ground.
- Gently thrust your elbows forward, parallel to the ground.
- Keep the rest of your body stationary.

Note: Sitting on a foam roller is not mandatory, but it does incorporate balance into the stretch.

Shoulder and Spine Twist

(Stretches: posterior deltoid, spine rotators, rhomboids, middle and lower trapezius)

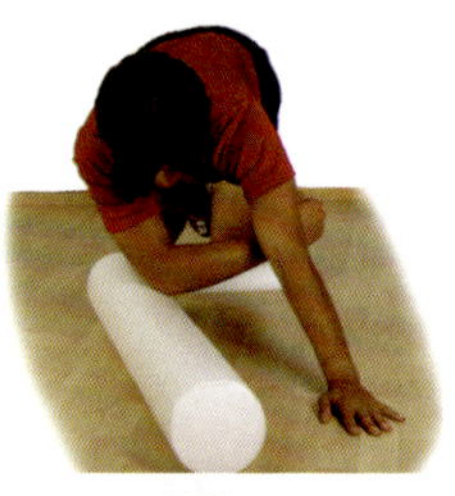

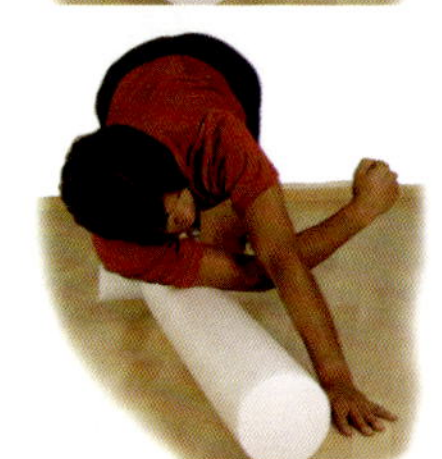

- Kneel on a half roller placed on the floor.
- Place a full roller on the floor and lean over it (as if you were going to do a push-up), so it runs length-wise along your body.
- Place your right elbow on the roller so your arm is behind your left arm.
- Brace yourself with your left arm.
- Lower your right shoulder so that your upper arm slides onto the roller.
- Hold for 30 to 60 seconds and repeat 2 to 3 times.
- Switch sides.

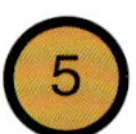

Behind the Back

(Stretches: anterior deltoid, chest, biceps)

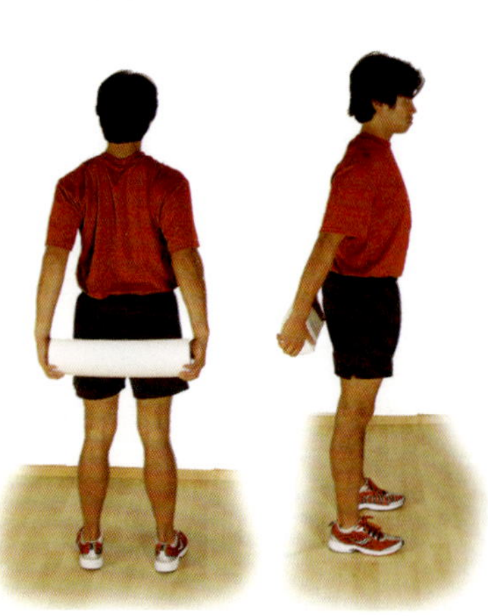

- Stand and hold a half roller at both ends, behind your back.
- Perform Girdle Grip (see pg. 8).
- Squeeze your shoulder blades back and down, and rotate your elbows around behind you.
- Keep your neck neutral as you look forward.
- Take a deep breath and feel your chest expand.
- Hold for 5 seconds and repeat 3 to 5 times.

Note: Common errors include rounding your shoulders, depressing your rib cage and poking your head forward.

6 Chair Arch

(Stretches: intercostals, pectoralis major, pectoralis minor, abdominals, arms down = plus anterior deltoid, biceps)

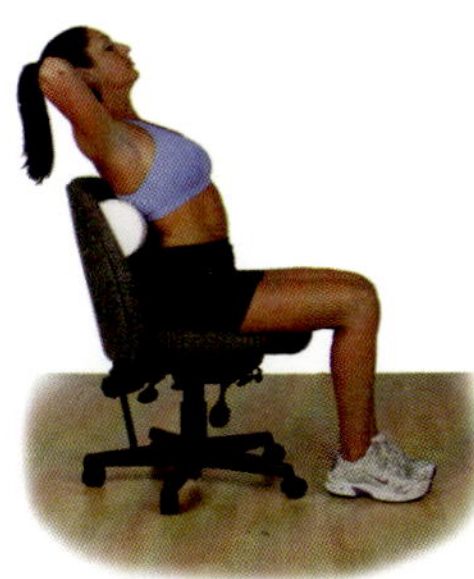

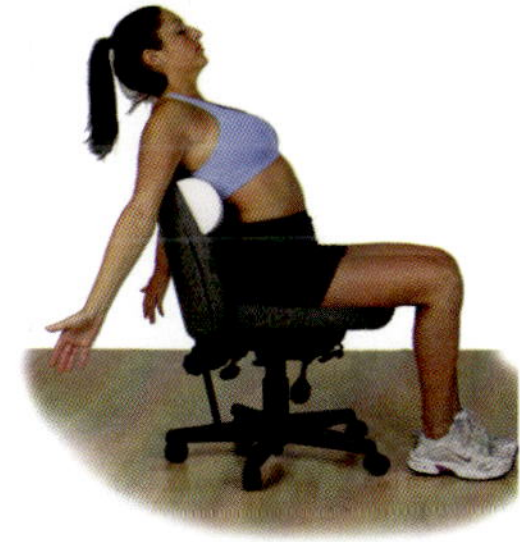

Arms Down

- Sit in a chair with a half roller placed across your mid-back.
- Place your hands behind your head, toward the top of your head.
- Perform Girdle Grip (see pg. 8).
- Squeeze your shoulder blades back and down. Open your chest to bring your elbows around behind your head.
- Keep your neck neutral and feet flat on the floor as you look slightly upward to the ceiling.
- Take a deep breath and feel your chest expand.
- Hold for 5 seconds and repeat 3 to 5 times.

Note: Those with excessive lower back arches, such as pregnant women, should not use a roller. Consult a professional for modifications.

Variation: Drop your arms down and behind your chair.

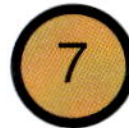

Chair Twists

(Stretches: spinal rotators, obliques, anterior deltoid)

- Sit on the front of your seat so your upper back is clear of the seat.
- Use your arms to secure a half roller against your mid-back.
- Perform Girdle Grip (pg. 8).
- Rotate your torso until you feel a comfortable stretch.
- Breathe deeply. As you exhale, twist a little more.
- Hold for 30 to 60 seconds and repeat 2 to 3 times. Switch sides.

Note: This stretch works best when you sit up straight.

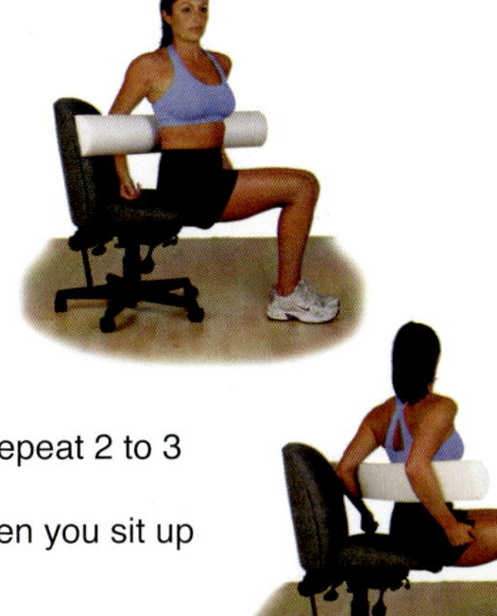

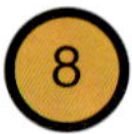

T-Spine Creeping

(Stretches: thoracic spine, rib cage, chest)

- Place a rolled towel or 12-inch water noodle (flotation toy) so it will run lengthwise along your upper mid-spine.
- Lay on the towel and rest your arms out to your sides at shoulder height.
- Relax in this position for 1 minute.
- Perform the Soreness Test (pg. 7).
- Over time build up to 5 minutes.

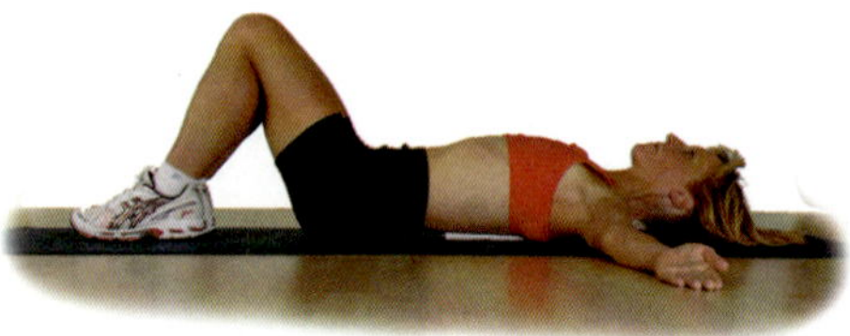

Note:

- This is best done at night, before bed, to help with relaxation.
- Don't force the spine: start with a short water noodle or towel.

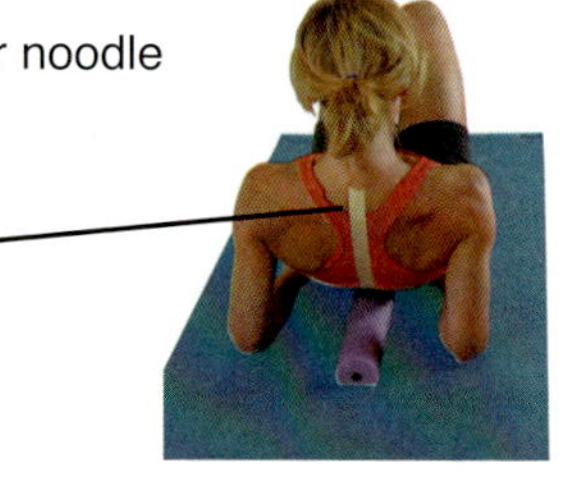

Tape shows thoracic spine

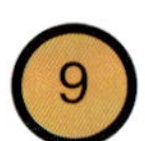

L-Spine Creeping

(Stretches: arch = lumbar spine, abdominals, rib cage, flatten = lumbar spine, erector spinae)

Choosing the right stretch

Arch Stretch: For those with a rounded lower back (slouched), such as when sitting all day:

- Lay on a half roller crosswise under your lower back. The arch should feel gentle and comfortable. Continue to Point "a" below.

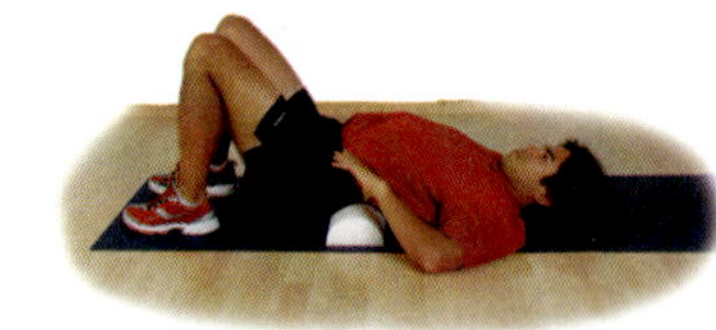

Arch stretch

Flatten Stretch: For those with an arched lower back (excessively lordotic), such as when pregnant or with a big belly:

- Lay on a half roller crosswise under your buttocks. The lower back should flatten against the floor, and feel gentle and comfortable. Continue to Point "a" below.

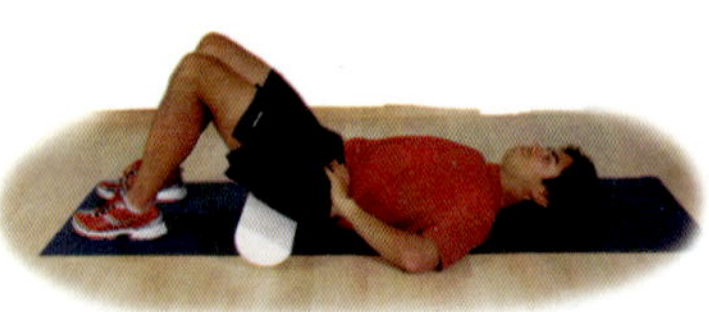

Flatten stretch

Next step for both Arch and Flatten

a. Relax in this position for 1 minute and then perform the Soreness Test (pg. 7).

b. Over time, build up to 5 minutes – pregnant women should never exceed 5 minutes.

c. Don't force the spine: start with a small roller or towel.

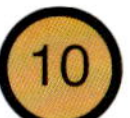

Double Knee-Lower Back

(Stretches: lumbar spine, erector spinae)

- Place a half roller on the floor, round side down, so it will run lengthwise along your spine.
- Lay on the roller and rest your arms out to your sides at shoulder height.
- Bend your knees and raise your legs onto a body ball, or simply place your feet flat on the floor.
- Keeping your feet together, gently lower your knees to the left until you feel a comfortable stretch.
- Pause in this position for 30 to 60 seconds.

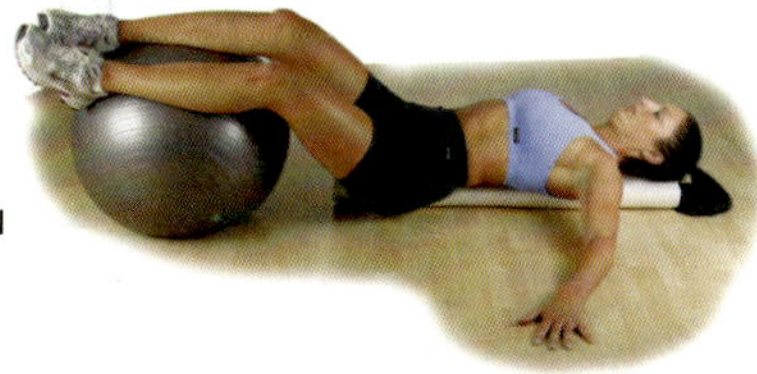

Back of the Thigh

(Stretches: hamstrings, toes back = plus gastrocnemius)

- Sit up straight on a chair, with a foam roller placed lengthwise along your spine.
- Raise your right leg straight in front of you, while keeping your foot relaxed and toes pointing forward.
- Contract your top thigh muscles to enhance the stretch on the back of the thigh. Switch sides.

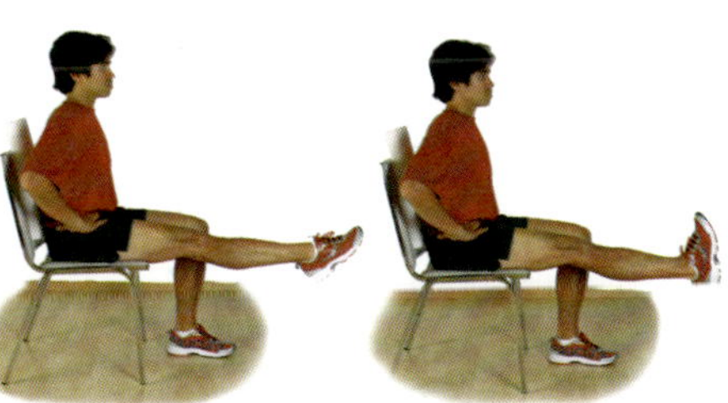

Toes forward *Toes back*

Progression:

- Keeping your spine straight and chest high, lean forward slightly.
- Extend your heel forward and pull your toes toward your shin.

Prone Quad and Hip Flexor

(Stretches: quadriceps, hip flexors)

- Lay face down and place a half roller crosswise under your right thigh, slightly above your knee.
- Place your left hand under your forehead to keep your neck and head aligned and comfortable.
- Bend your right leg.
- Grab your right ankle with your right hand and pull your heel toward your buttocks.
- Squeeze your buttocks and press your pelvis into the floor.
- Do not arch your lower back.
- Switch sides.

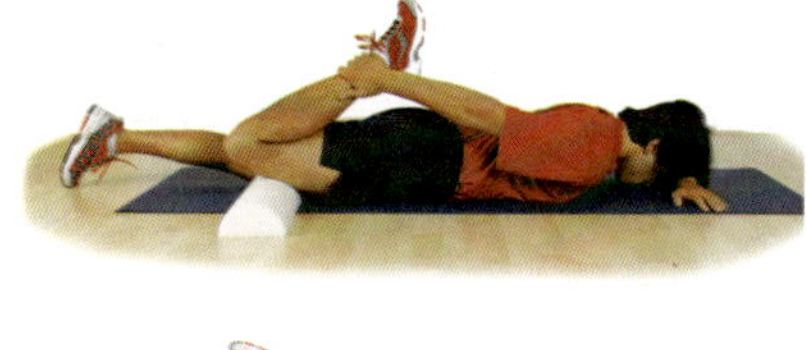

Modification:

Wrap a towel or belt around your ankle to extend your reach – but never stretch to the point of pain.

Deep Buttocks and Hip

(Stretches: piriformis)

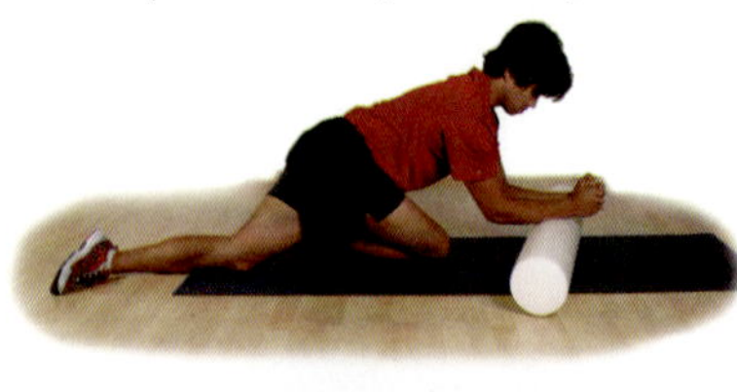

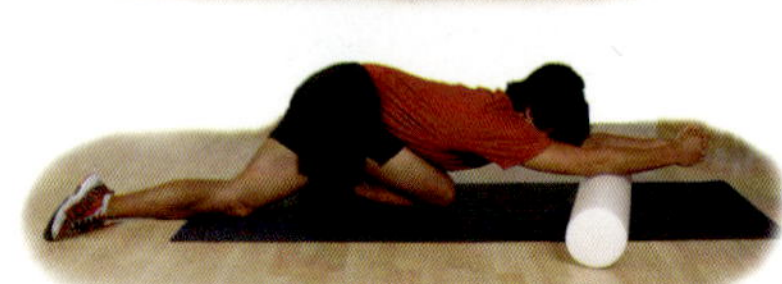

- Kneel and place your forearms on a foam roller.
- Lift your left leg over your right leg and straighten it out.
- Then gently slide your left leg toward a five o'clock position.
- At the same time, sit down onto your right heel.
- Roll your arms forward on the roller, and gently drop your left shoulder.
- Switch sides.

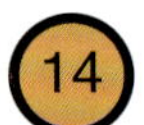

Bent-Knee Calf Stretch

(Stretches: toes up = soleus, toes down = tibialis anterior)

- Sit on a chair and place your feet on a half roller.
- Slowly lower your heels to the floor.
- Pull your toes toward your shins to increase the stretch.
- Push your toes down to stretch the front of your shin.

Note: In the workplace, place the roller under your desk and keep your heels down while you work.

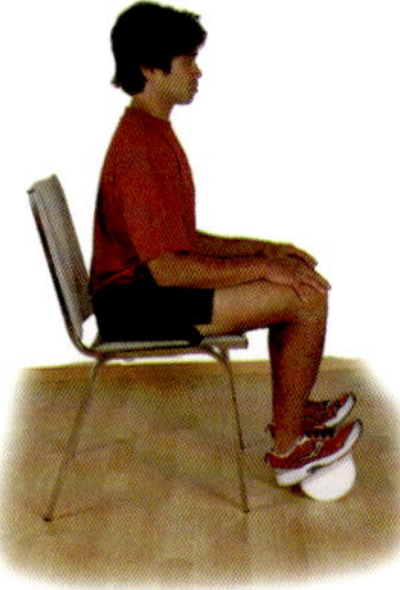

Toes up

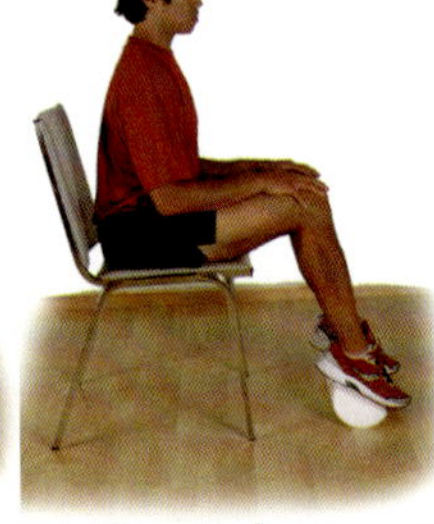

Toes down

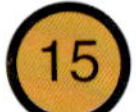

Straight-knee Calf Stretch

(Stretches: gastrocnemius Variation: back leg = gastrocnemius, front leg = soleus)

- Stand with both feet on a half roller and support your balance with a desk, roller or other support structure.
- Slowly lower your heels to the floor.
- Pull your toes toward your shins to increase the stretch.

Variation:

- Leave your left leg on the roller and step back with the right leg.
- Straighten your right leg, gradually pushing your heel to the floor.
- Stop when you feel a comfortable stretch in the right calf.
- Pull your toes toward your shins to increase the stretch in your calves. Switch sides.

Note:

- Keep your heels on the floor.

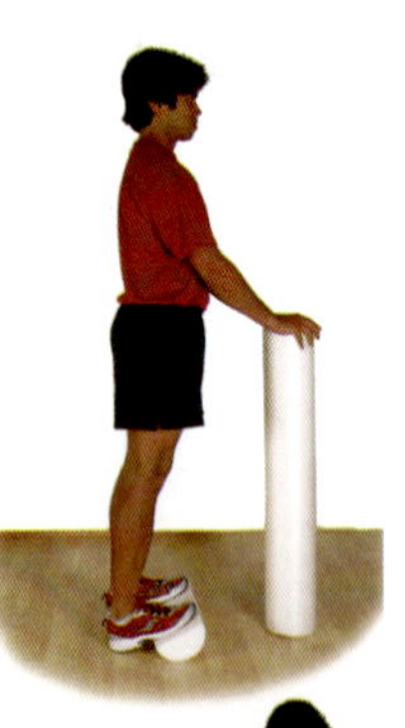

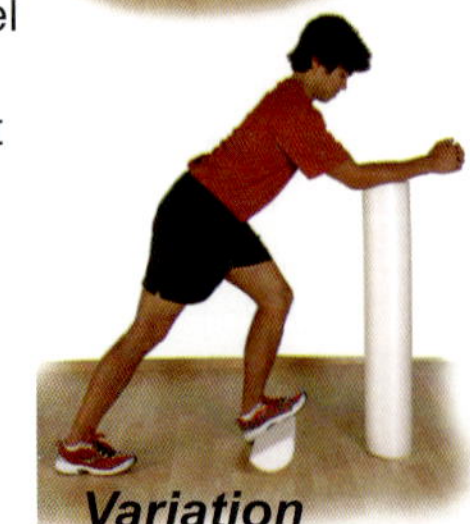

Variation

STANDING EXERCISES

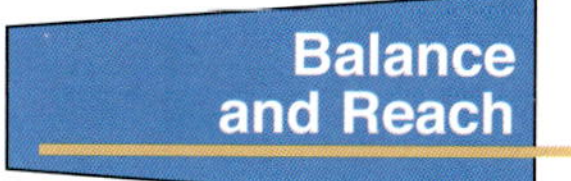

Muscles worked: neck retractors, erector spinae, deltoid, anatomical girdle, postural hip and ankle stabilizers

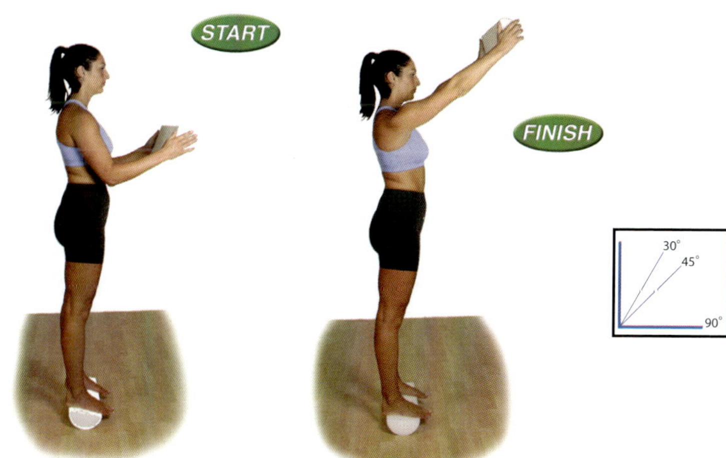

Hold 5 seconds

1. Stand on a half roller (as shown) with your feet hip-width apart and knees slightly bent.
2. Imagine a broomstick against your spine.
3. Perform the Girdle Grip (pg. 8).
4. Holding a half roller, bend and raise your arms to a 45° angle.
5. Keep your shoulder blades back and down.
6. Hold for 5 seconds with your arms raised in the air while maintaining your balance.
7. Repeat 5 times.

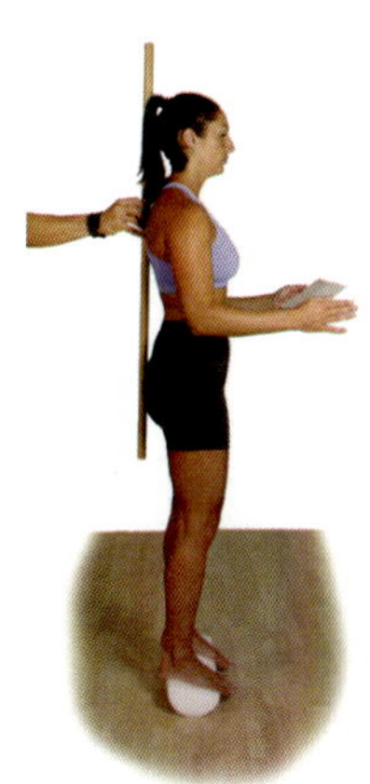

Progression:
1. Build up to 1-minute holds for 2 sets.
2. Add 2 to 5 pound dumbbells.
3. Add small 3-inch arm movements, such as circles and up/down movements.

Balance and Turn

Muscles worked: neck retractors, erector spinae, deltoid, anatomical girdle, postural hip and ankle stabilizers

1. Stand on a half roller with your feet hip-width apart.
2. Perform the Girdle Grip (pg. 8) and stand tall.
3. Holding a short foam roller between your hands, raise your arms straight out in front of you.
4. Keep your shoulder blades back and down.
5. While maintaining your balance, slowly turn your torso to the right.
7. Pause and hold for 5 seconds.
8. Switch sides.
9. Build up to 1-minute arm holds, while maintaining your balance.

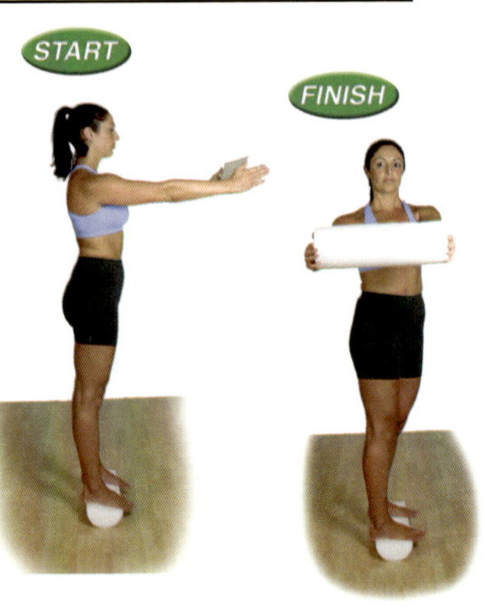

Variation:
Lift your arms to a 45° angle.

30° 45° 90°

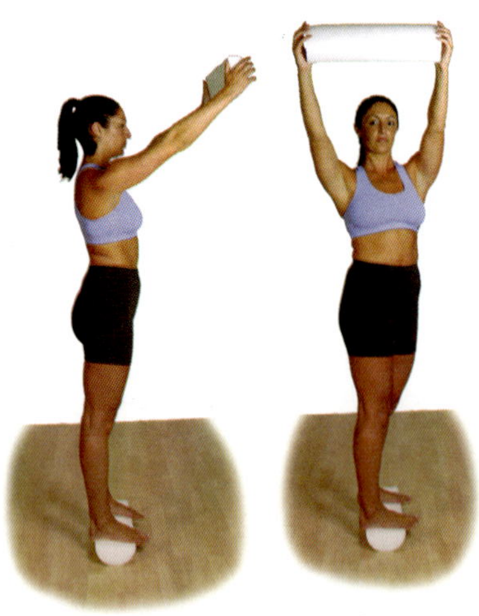

Hold 5 seconds

Progression:
1. Add 2 to 5 pound dumbbells.
2. Add small 3-inch arm movements, such as circles and up/down movements.

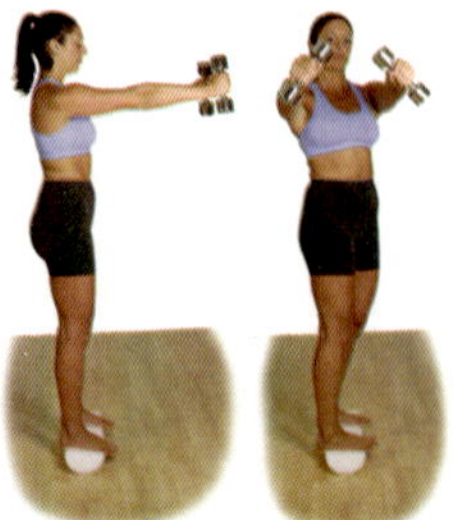

Hold 5 seconds

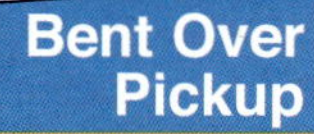

Bent Over Pickup

Muscles worked: neck retractors, erector spinae, deltoid, anatomical girdle, hip extensors, ankle stabilizers

Standing

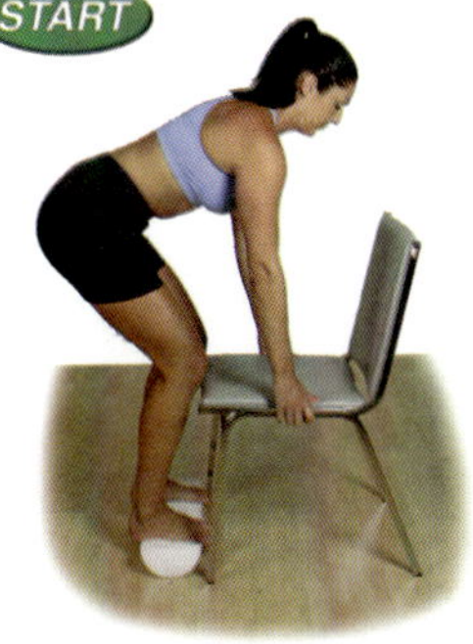

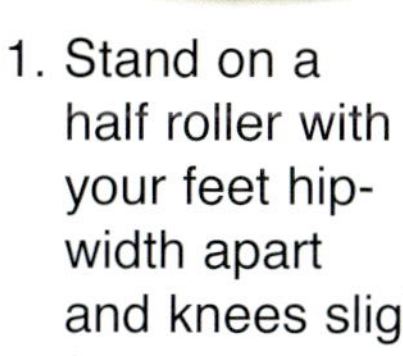

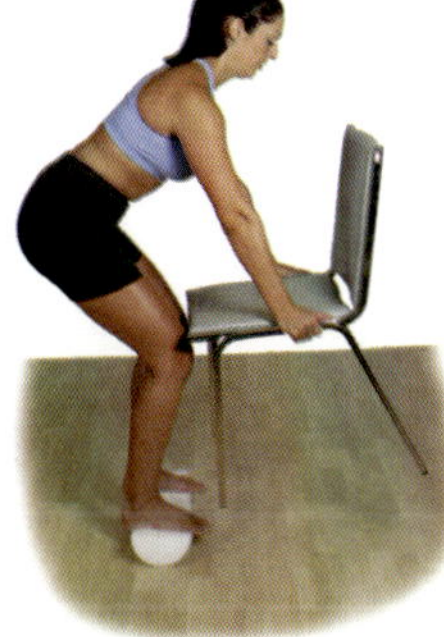

Hold 5 seconds

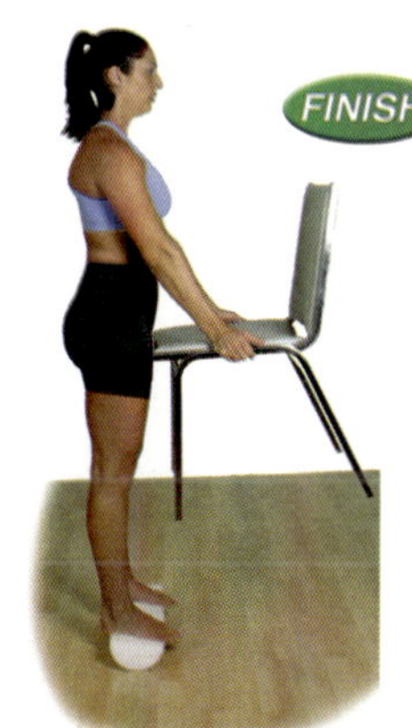

Hold 5 seconds

1. Stand on a half roller with your feet hip-width apart and knees slightly bent, directly in front of a chair.
2. Perform the Girdle Grip (pg. 8). Imagine a broomstick against your spine. Keep a slight arch in your back and concentrate on maintaining proper posture as you reach down.
3. Slowly lift the chair off the ground while maintaining your balance and posture. Keep the chair close to your legs as you lift. Hold the bent over position for 5 seconds.
4. Bring yourself to a standing position and hold for 5 seconds.
5. In the same controlled fashion, place the chair back on the floor.
6. Repeat 5 times.

Progression:

1. Build up to 1-minute holds.

Variation: Bent Over Turn and Pick-Up

1. Hold a dumbbell (vertically) between your thighs.
2. Turn to the left, squat and bend forward slightly.
3. Hold this position for 5 seconds.
4. Then stand up straight and face forward.
5. Turn to the right, squat and bend forward slightly.

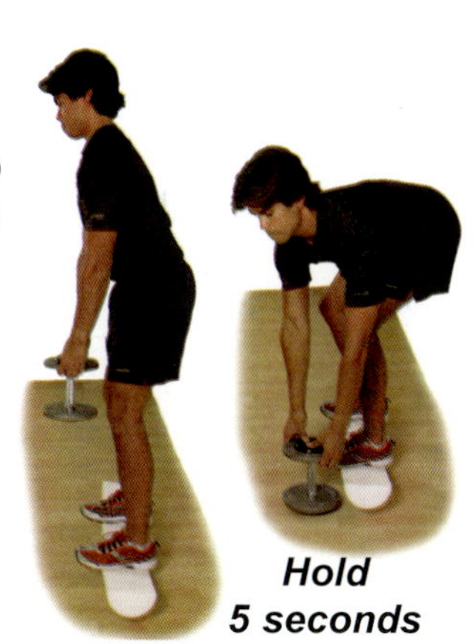

Hold 5 seconds

Front Squat

Muscles worked: neck retractors, scapular retractors, erector spinae, deltoid, anatomical girdle, hip extensors, quadriceps, ankle stabilizers

1. Place a half roller on the floor, 5 inches from a wall.
2. Stand on the half roller with your toes about 3 inches from the wall. You may have to adjust the roller's position relative to the wall.
3. Place a broomstick behind your head so it rests on your upper back muscles, (NOT THE SPINE).
4. Perform the Girdle Grip (pg. 8) and stand tall.
5. Look slightly downwards.
6. Squat down slightly so that your buttocks stick out, as if you are going to sit in a chair. Don't tuck your buttocks under you.
7. Keep your shoulder blades back and down, and your chest high.
8. Bend forward from the hips approximately 30° to 45° - but maintain a neutral straight spine (imagine a stick on your back).
9. Hold this position for 5 seconds and then stand up straight. Repeat 5 times.

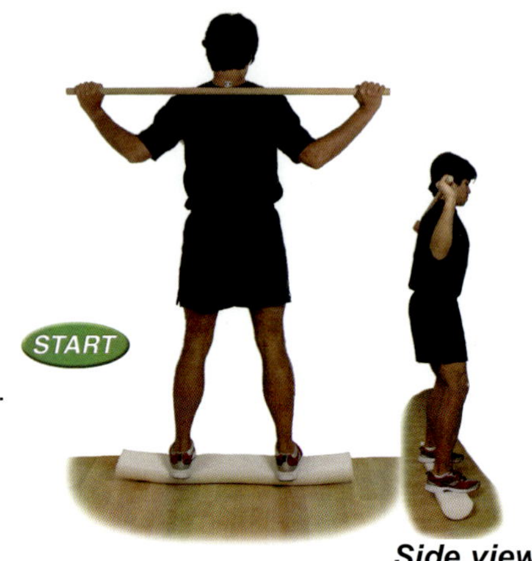

Side view

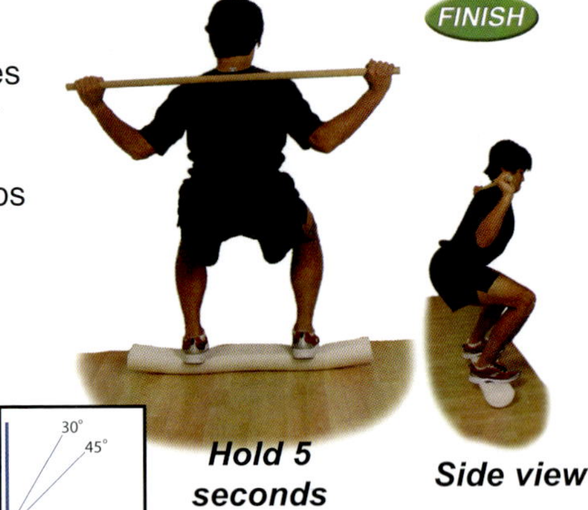

Hold 5 seconds

Side view

Note:

Don't poke your head forward; bend forward at the hips instead, and arch your back like a ski ramp.

Progression:

1. Build up to 1-minute holds.
2. While in the down position, shift your pelvis from side to side.
3. Also in the down position, rock your feet back and forth without losing balance.
4. Replace the broomstick for a barbell or body toning bar.

Adv. Overhead Press Squat

Muscles worked: neck retractors, scapular retractors, erector spinae, deltoid, anatomical girdle, postural hip and ankle stabilizers

1. Place a half roller on the floor, 5 inches from a wall.
2. Stand on the half roller with your toes about 3 inches from the wall. You may have to adjust the roller's position relative to the wall.
3. Raise a broomstick over your head, with your palms facing the wall and your hands 3 to 4 feet apart.
4. Perform the Girdle Grip (pg. 8) and stand tall.
5. Look slightly downwards.
6. Squat down slightly so that your buttocks stick out, as if you are going to sit in a chair. Don't tuck your buttocks under you.
7. Keep your shoulder blades back and down, and your chest high. Do not let anything touch the wall.
8. Bend forward from the hips approximately 30° to 45° - but maintain a neutral straight spine (imagine a stick on your back).
9. Hold this position for 5 seconds and then stand up straight. Repeat 5 times.

Note:

It is normal to feel a great amount of muscular work in your back muscles.

Progression:

1. Build up to 1-minute holds.
2. While in the down position, shift your pelvis from side to side.
3. Also in the down position, rock your feet back and forth without losing balance.
4. Replace the broomstick for a barbell or body toning bar.
5. Use a full, circular roller.

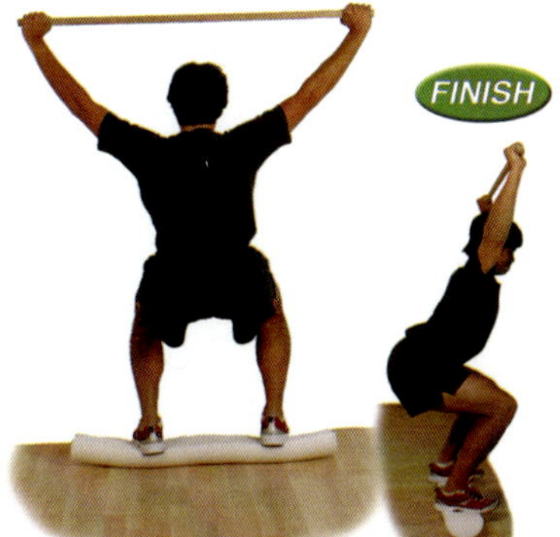

Hold 5 seconds ***Side view***

Samurai

Muscles worked: erector spinae, spinal rotators, neck rotators, deltoid, external rotator cuff

Standing

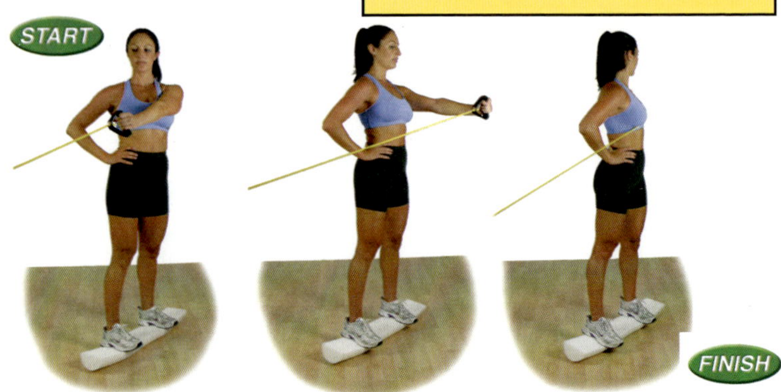

1. Anchor an exercise stretch tube at mid-waist height.
2. Stand on a half roller perpendicular to the anchor point, far enough away to stretch the tubing taut.
3. Ensure your feet are hip-width apart, facing away from the anchor point. Place your right hand on your hip bone.
4. Grip the tube handle with your left hand. Lift your arm straight out in front.
5. Perform the Girdle Grip (pg. 8) and stand tall.
6. Release some slack by turning your upper body and arm to the right while keeping your hips facing forward.
7. Slowly pull the tubing to the left, across the front of your body, with a straight arm, and hold for 5 seconds.
8. Repeat 8 to 12 times. Then switch sides.

Variations:

1. Attach tubing high and pull high to low.

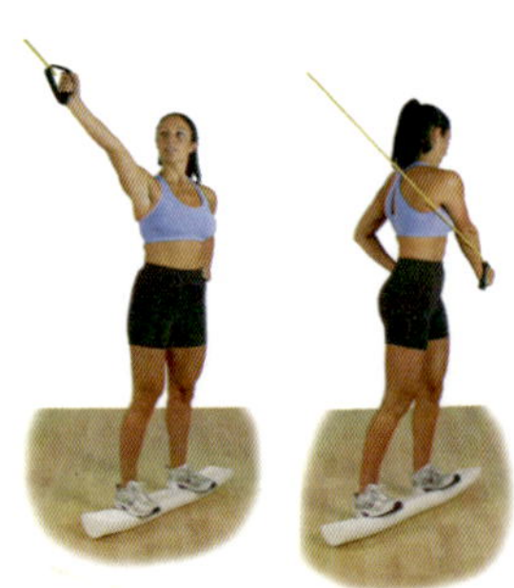

Note:

1. Maintain solid torso stability throughout the movement.
2. Let the arm, shoulder and spine do the work.

Samurai Double Arm

Muscles worked: erector spinae, spinal rotators, deltoid, chest, abdominals

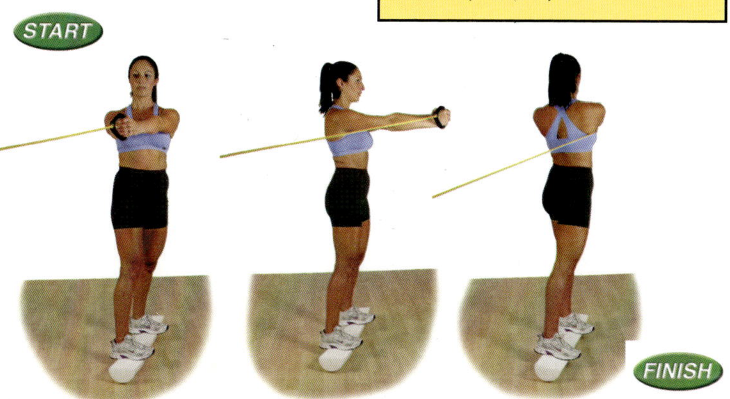

1. Anchor an exercise stretch tube at mid-waist height.
2. Stand on a half roller perpendicular to the anchor point, far enough away to stretch the tubing taut.
3. Ensure your feet are hip-width apart, facing away from the anchor point.
4. Grip the tube handle with both hands. Lift your arms straight out in front.
5. Perform the Girdle Grip (pg. 8) and stand tall.
6. Release some slack by turning your upper body and arm to the right while keeping your hips facing forward.
7. Slowly pull the tubing to the left, across the front of your body, with straight arms, and hold for 5 seconds.
8. Repeat 8 to 12 times. Then switch sides.

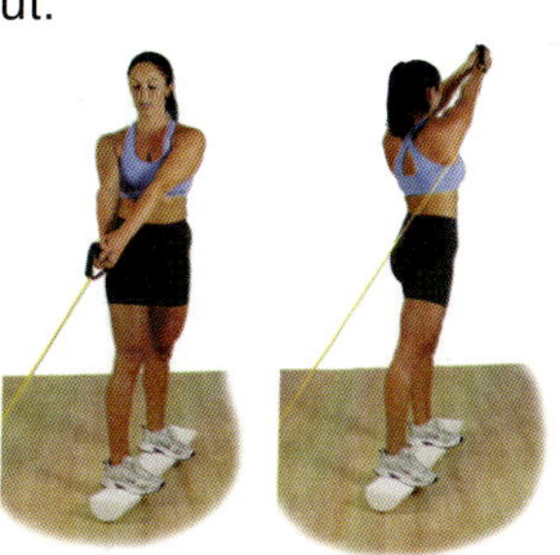

Variations:

1. Attach tubing high and pull high to low.
2. Attach tubing low and pull low to high.

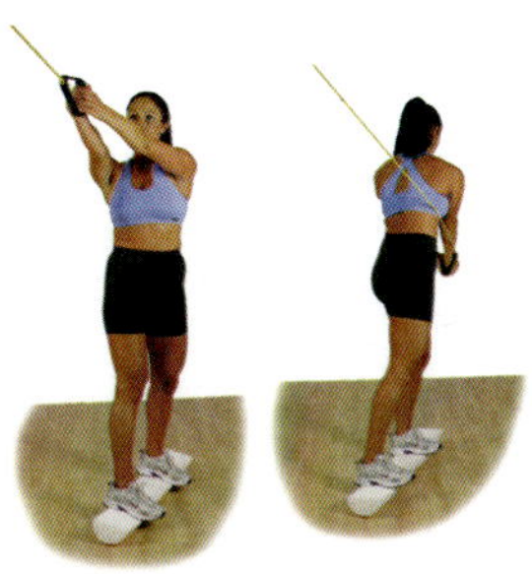

Note:

1. Maintain solid torso stability throughout the movement.
2. Let the arm, shoulder and spine do the work.

Split Squat

Muscles worked: abdominals, chest, quadriceps, adductors, hip flexors (back leg), hip extensors (front leg), spinal rotators, deltoid, external rotator cuff

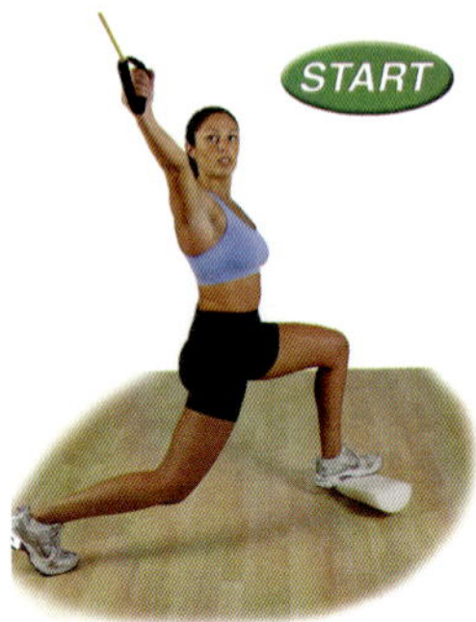

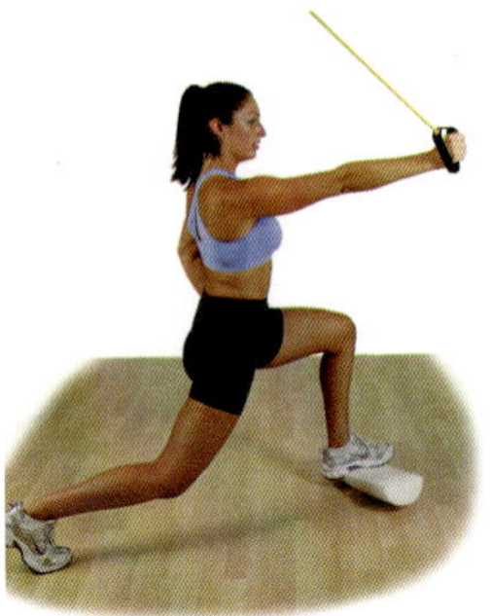

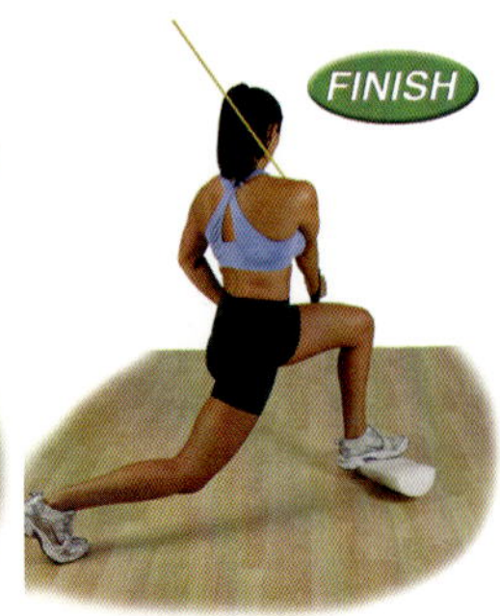

1. Anchor an exercise stretch tube at head height.
2. Place your left foot on a half roller, far enough away to stretch the tubing taut.
3. Grip the tube handle with your right hand. Lift your arm straight out in front.
4. Step your right foot backwards by 2 to 3 feet. Place your left hand on your hip bone.
5. Perform the Girdle Grip (pg. 8) and stand tall.
6. With your feet in place, slowly lower your body by bending at the knees, keeping your torso upright and front knee at 90°. Turn your upper body and arm to the right, in line with the direction of the tubing.
7. Slowly pull the tubing to the left, down and across the front of your body, with a straight arm, and hold for 5 seconds.
8. Repeat 8 to 12 times. Then switch sides.

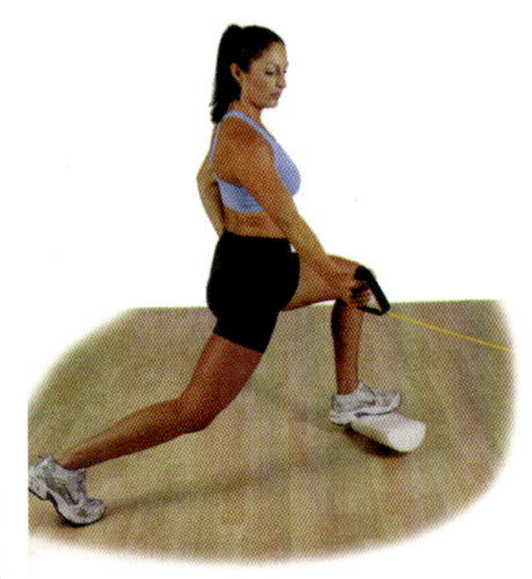

Variations:

1. Attach tubing low and pull low to high.

Note:

1. Maintain solid torso stability throughout the movement.
2. Let the arm, shoulder and spine do the work.

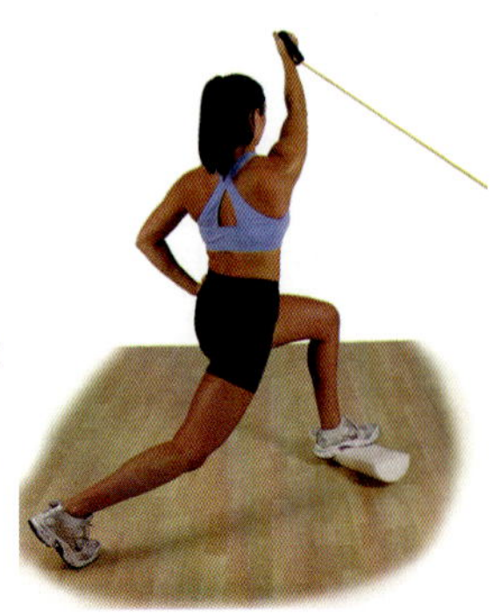

Sitting EXERCISES

Posture with Shoulders

Muscles worked: neck retractors, erector spinae, deltoid, anatomical girdle, postural stabilizers

START

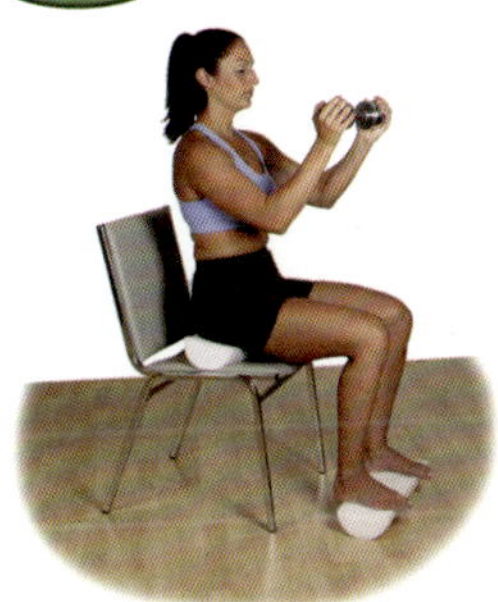

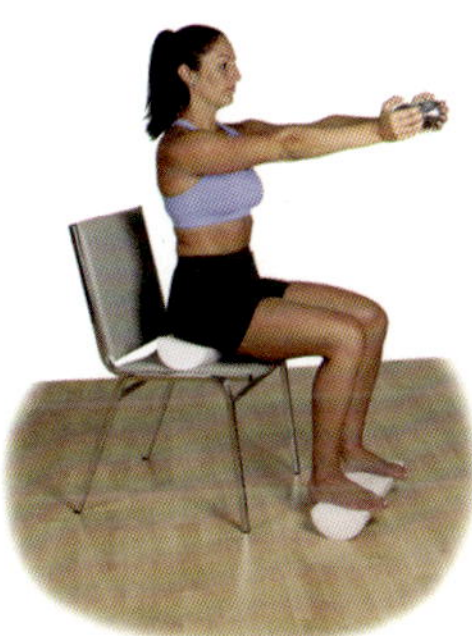

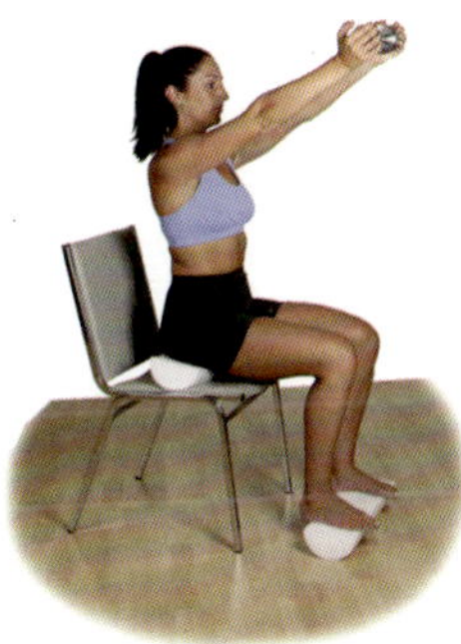

FINISH

1. Sit on a half roller placed across a seat. Place your feet hip-width apart on a half roller, or on the floor.
2. Grip a dumbbell with both hands, by the ends.
3. Perform the Girdle Grip (pg. 8) and sit up tall. Imagine a broomstick against your spine.
4. Slowly straighten your arms, holding the dumbbell directly out in front of you.
5. Now slowly raise your arms to a 45° angle.
6. Keep your shoulder blades back and down.
7. Hold for 5 seconds and repeat 5 times.

30° 45° 90°

Note: Don't lean backwards, reduce the weight lifted instead.

Progression:

1. Build up to 1-minute holds for 2 sets.
2. Build up to 2 to 5 pound dumbbells.

Variation:

Holding a dumbbell in each hand, alternate straightening your arms.

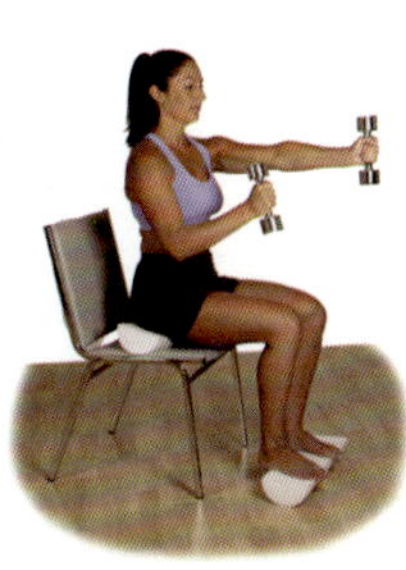

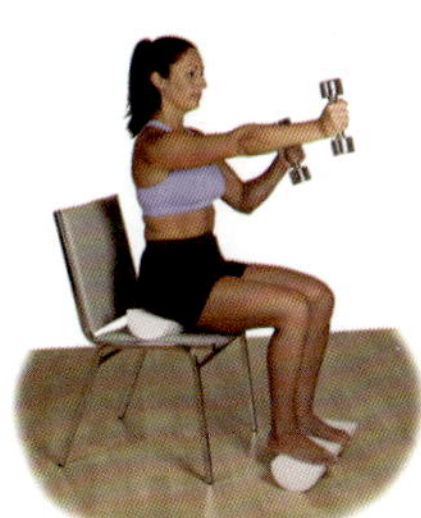

Sit, Twist and Hold

Muscles worked: neck retractors, erector spinae, spinal rotators, deltoid, anatomical girdle, postural stabilizers

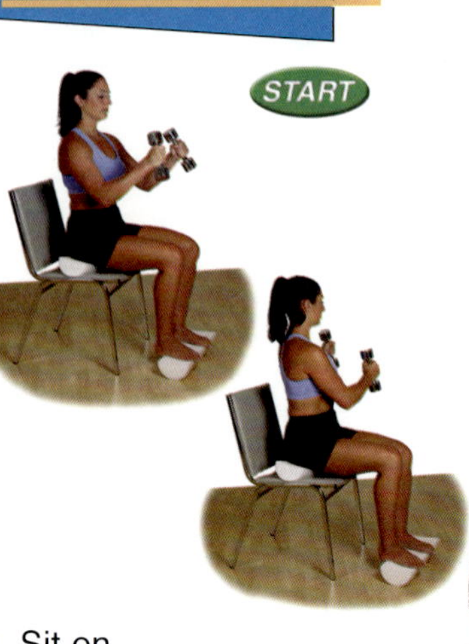

1. Sit on a half roller placed across a seat. Place your feet hip-width apart on a half roller, or on the floor.
2. Grip a dumbbell in each hand.
3. Perform the Girdle Grip (pg. 8).
4. Rotate your torso to the left and gently punch out with your right hand and hold for 5 seconds.
5. Return to center and then turn your torso to the right.
6. Gently punch out with your left hand. Keep your shoulder blades back and down.
7. Hold for 5 seconds and repeat 5 times.

Note: Don't lean backwards; reduce the weight lifted instead.

Progression:

1. Build up to 1-minute holds for 2 sets.
2. Increase the dumbbell weight.

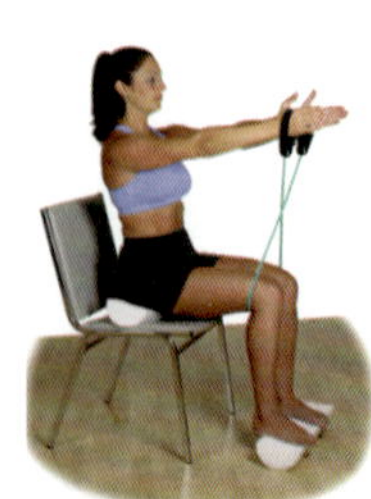

Variation with tubing

Leaning Torso

Muscles worked: neck retractors, erector spinae, deltoid, anatomical girdle, hip extensors, postural stabilizers, **Advanced Variation** = plus scapular stabilizers, lower trapezius

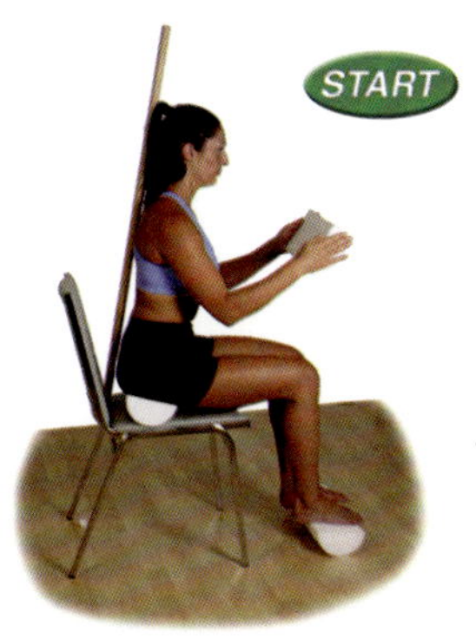

Note: The broomstick is only to show proper posture. It is not required for the exercise.

1. Sit on a half roller placed across a seat. Place your feet hip-width apart on a half roller, or on the floor.
2. Grip a roller with both hands, by the ends.
3. Perform the Girdle Grip (pg. 8) and sit up tall. Imagine a broomstick against your spine.
4. Lean your torso slightly forward without compromising posture.
5. Now slowly straighten your arms in front of you.
6. Keep your shoulder blades back and down.
7. Hold for 5 seconds and repeat 5 times.

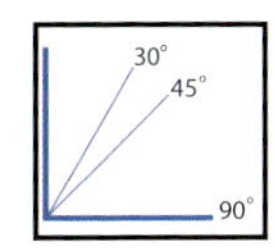

Progression:

1. Build up to 1-minute holds for 2 sets.
2. Raise your arms to a 45° angle.
3. Raise your arms to your ears (hardest).
4. Lift dumbbells instead of a roller.

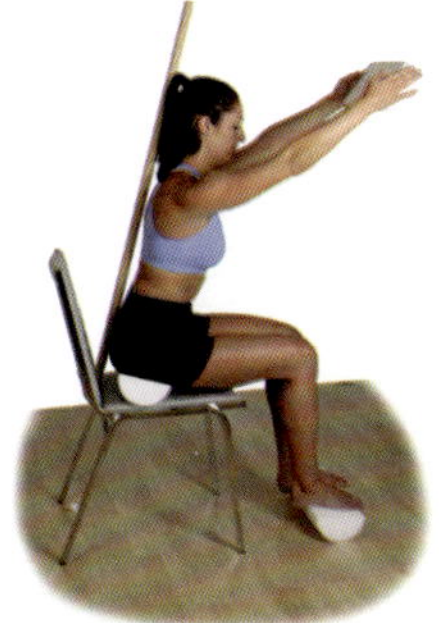

Variation at 45° angle

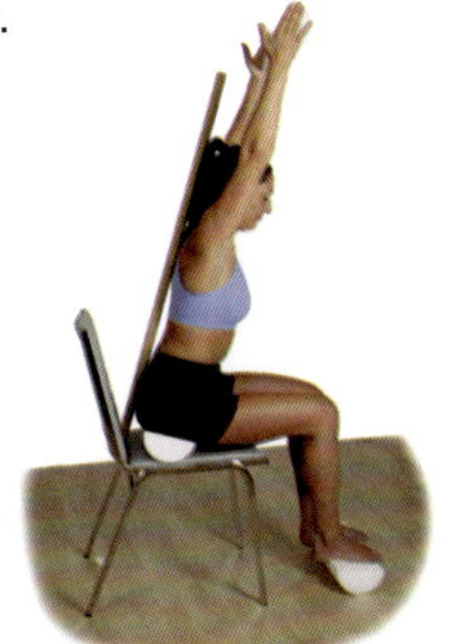

Advanced Variation with arms at ears

Leaning Torso Twist & Rotate

Muscles worked: neck retractors, erector spinae, deltoid, spinal rotators, anatomical girdle, hip extensors, postural stabilizers, scapular stabilizers

START

This is an advanced exercise

FINISH

1. Sit on a half roller placed across a seat. Place your feet hip-width apart on a half roller, or on the floor.

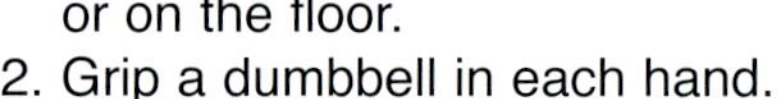

2. Grip a dumbbell in each hand.
3. Perform the Girdle Grip (pg. 8) and sit up tall. Imagine a broomstick against your spine.
4. Slowly lean forward and straighten your arms in front of you. Maintain proper posture throughout.
5. Keeping your arms extended, rotate your shoulders to the right and hold for 5 seconds.
6. Keep your shoulder blades back and down.
7. Return to center and rotate your shoulders to the left and hold for 5 seconds.

Progression:

1. Build up to 1-minute holds for 2 sets.
2. Increase the dumbbell weight.

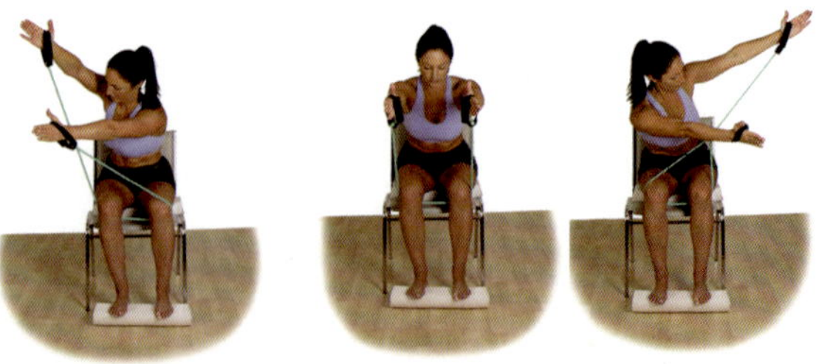

Variation:

Use stretch tubing secured at the back of your knees.

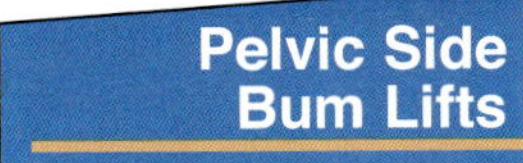

Pelvic Side Bum Lifts

Muscles worked: erector spinae, quadratus lumborum, obliques, anatomical girdle, postural stabilizers

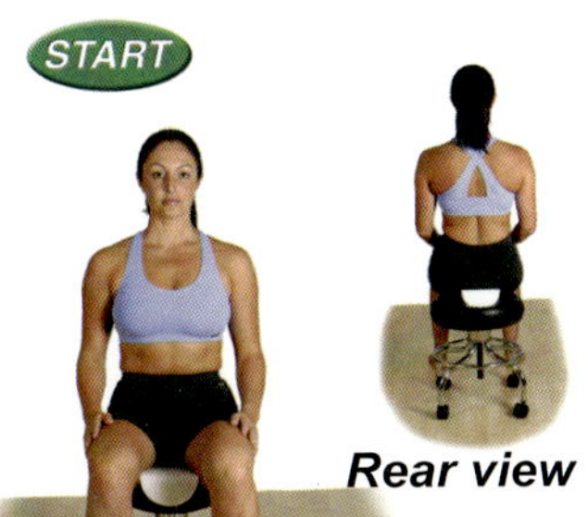

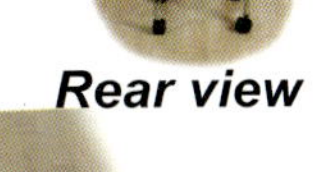
Rear view

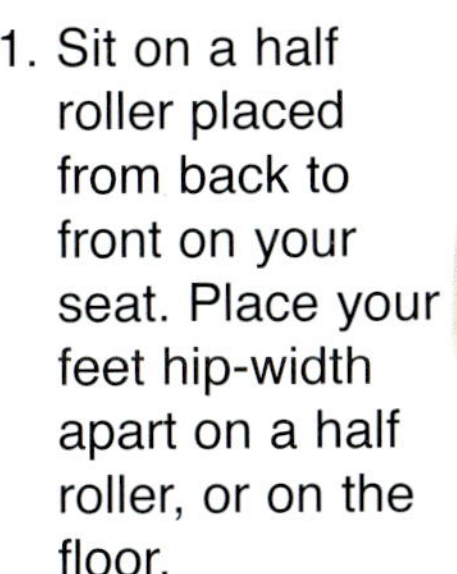

1. Sit on a half roller placed from back to front on your seat. Place your feet hip-width apart on a half roller, or on the floor.
2. Perform the Girdle Grip (pg. 8) and sit up tall. Imagine a broomstick against your spine.

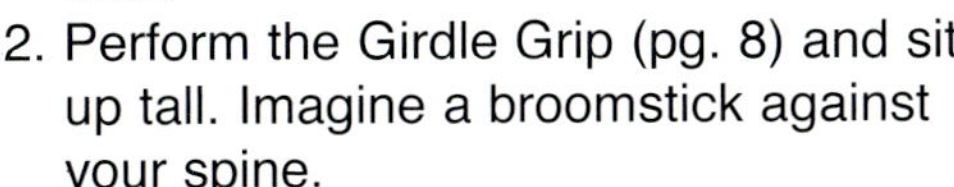

3. Slowly tilt your pelvis to the left and hold for 5 seconds.
4. Return to center.
5. Slowly tilt your pelvis to the right and hold for 5 seconds.
6. Keep your shoulder blades back and down.

FINISH

Progression:

1. Build up to 1-minute holds for 2 sets.

On Hands and Knees EXERCISES

1/2 Push Up

Muscles worked: neck retractors, chest, triceps, anatomical girdle, pelvis and hip stabilizers

START

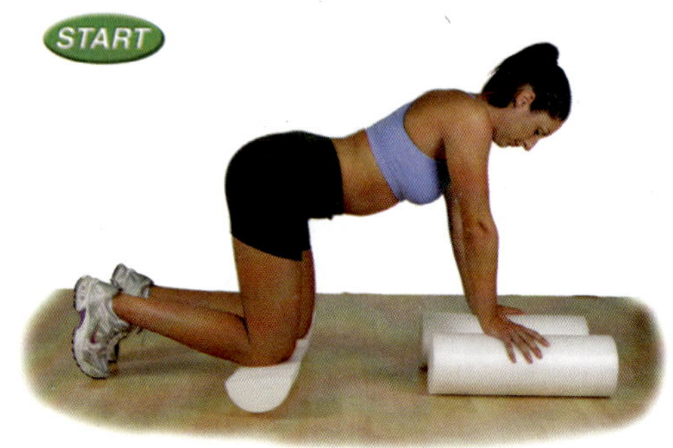

FINISH

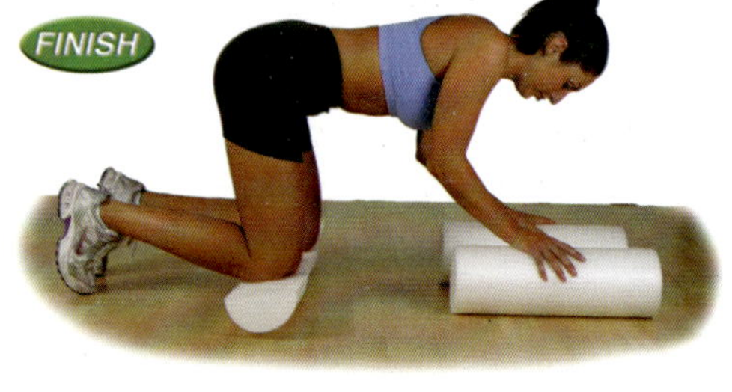

1. Kneel on a half roller.
2. Place a full or half roller lengthwise under each hand.
3. Perform the Girdle Grip (pg. 8). Imagine a broomstick against your spine.
4. Bend your arms and lower your upper body to comfortable and controlled position.
5. Hold for 5 seconds and then push up to the top position.
6. Repeat 5 times.

Progression:
1. Increase to 12 repetitions of 5-second holds at the bottom position.
2. Increase the distance between your hands and knees.
3. Finally, move from your knees to your feet (still balancing on a half roller), and perform a full push-up.

Baby Crawl

Muscles worked: neck extensors, latissimus dorsi, chest, triceps, anatomical girdle, pelvis and hip stabilizers

START

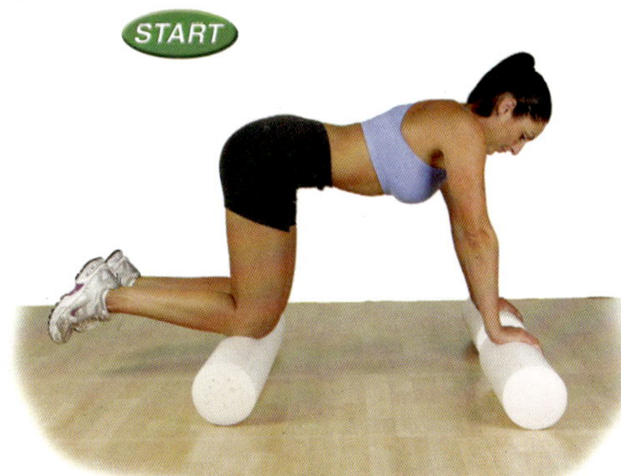

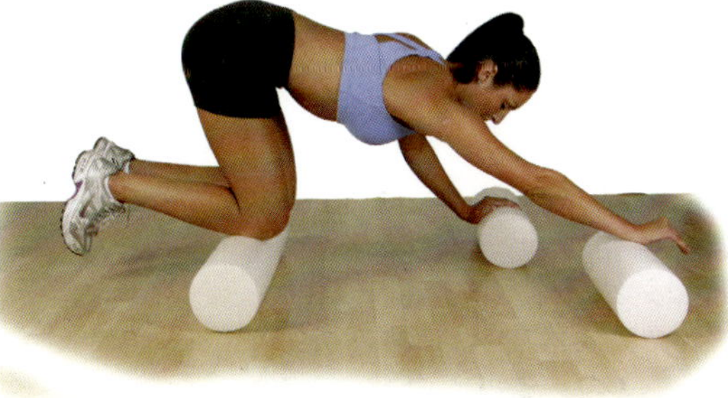

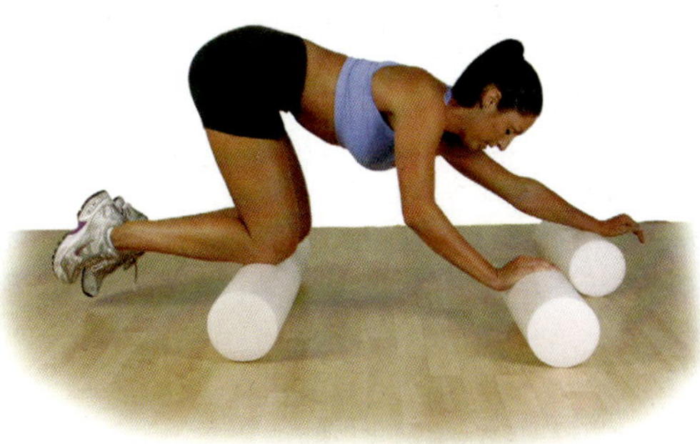

1. Kneel on a full roller (or half roller for more support).
2. Place a short roller under each hand.
3. Perform the Girdle Grip (pg. 8). Imagine a broomstick against your spine.
4. Maintaining your balance and your posture, roll forward with your right hand, supporting your weight on both front rollers.
5. Roll forward 6 to 8 inches and hold for 5 seconds.
6. Return to the starting position and then roll forward with the left hand.
7. Remember to breathe rhythmically.
8. Repeat 5 times on each side.

Leg Lift

Muscles worked: neck retractors, erector spinae, spine, anatomical girdle, pelvis and hip stabilizers, hip extensors

START

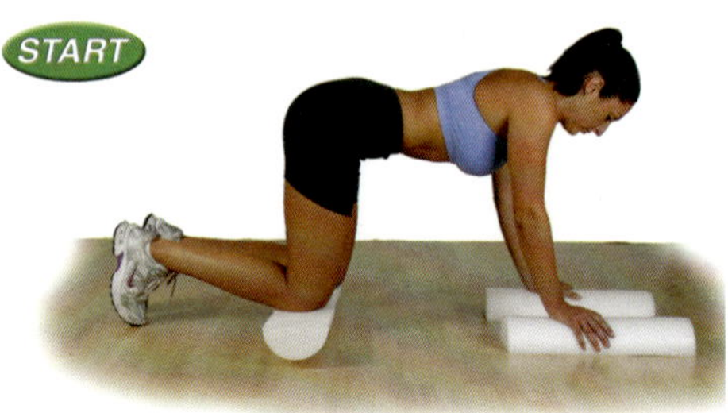

1. Kneel on a half roller, round side down.
2. Place a full or half roller lengthwise under each hand.
3. Perform the Girdle Grip (pg. 8). Imagine a broomstick against your spine.
4. Bend your right leg and lift it behind you until your thigh is parallel to the ground.
5. Then straighten your right leg – but keep your thigh parallel to the ground.
6. Hold this position for 5 seconds and then return to the starting position.
7. Repeat 5 times and switch sides.

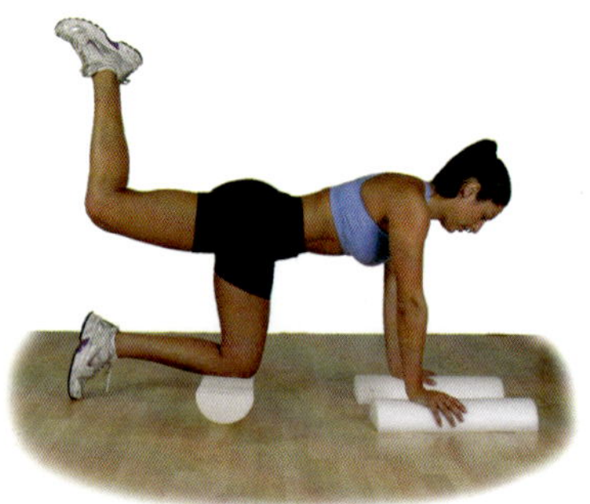

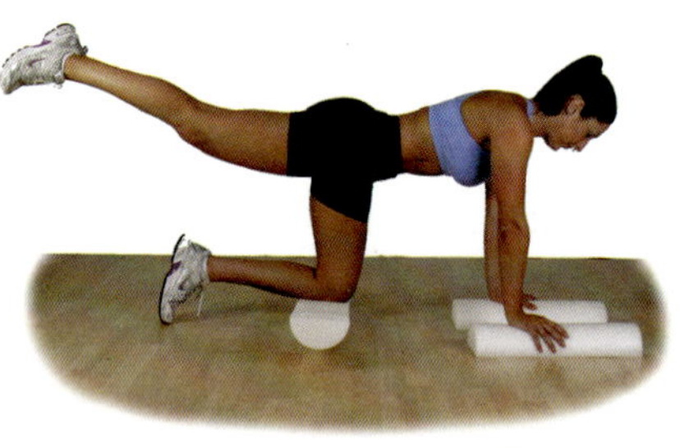

FINISH

Note:

1. Do not bend your arms or drop your thigh below parallel.
2. Do not sit back on your heels.

Progression:

1. Increase to 12 repetitions with 5-second holds.
2. Turn the half rollers under your hands so the round side faces down.

Half Superman

Muscles worked: neck retractors, deltoid, low trapezius, erector spinae, spine, anatomical girdle, pelvis and hip stabilizers, hip extensors

Variation: plus scapular retractors and hip abductors

1. Kneel on a half roller, round side down.
2. Place a full or half roller lengthwise under each hand.
3. Perform the Girdle Grip (pg. 8). Imagine a broomstick against your spine.
4. Raise your right arm and left leg slightly off the rollers.
5. Slowly and simultaneously begin raising and straightening your arm and leg.
6. Continue until your arm and leg are straight and are in line with your back.
7. Hold for 5 seconds. Then bring your right elbow and left knee together until they touch.
8. Repeat 5 times and switch sides.

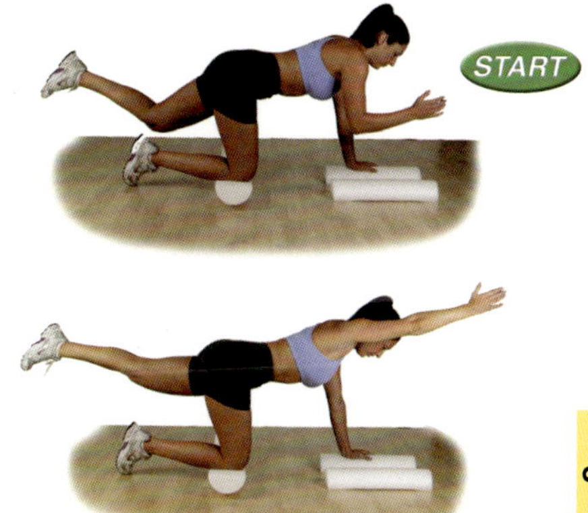

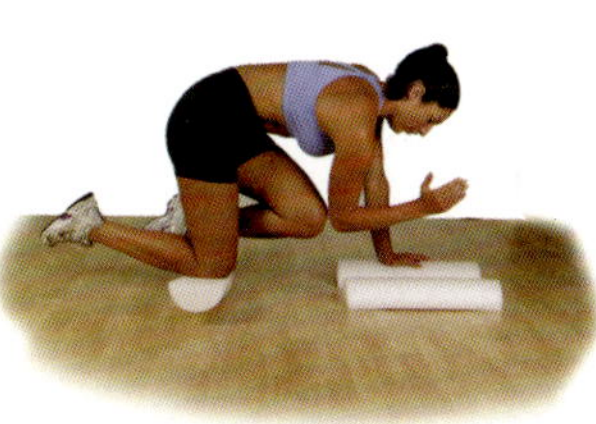

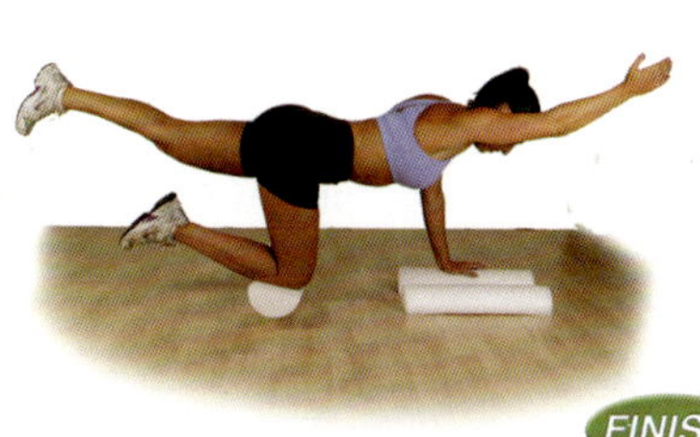

Variation:

1. Lift your arm and leg out to the side. Pause when they are parallel to the floor. Hold for 5 seconds.

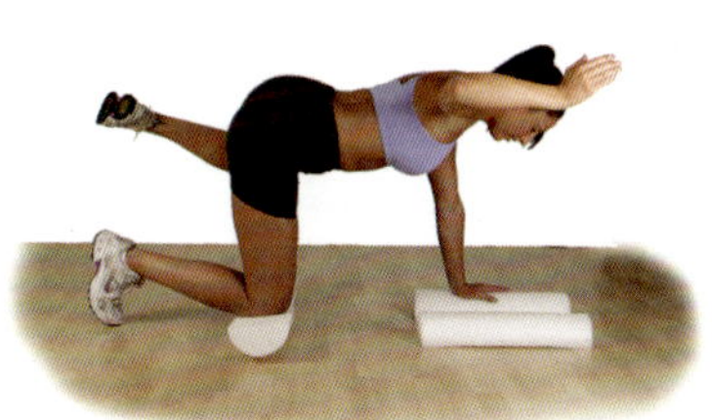

Elbow Walk

Muscles worked: neck retractors, deltoid, shoulder stabilizers, erector spinae, anatomical girdle, pelvis and hip stabilizers

1. Kneel on a half roller and place your hands on either side of a short roller laid crosswise in front of you.
2. As you lean on your hands, keep your elbows straight.
3. Bend your left elbow and place it on the short roller.
4. Then bend your right elbow and also place it on the roller.
5. Place your left hand on the floor, back to its starting position, with elbow straight.
6. Then place your right hand on the floor, also back in its starting position.
7. Repeat 4 to 6 full cycles of this "walk".

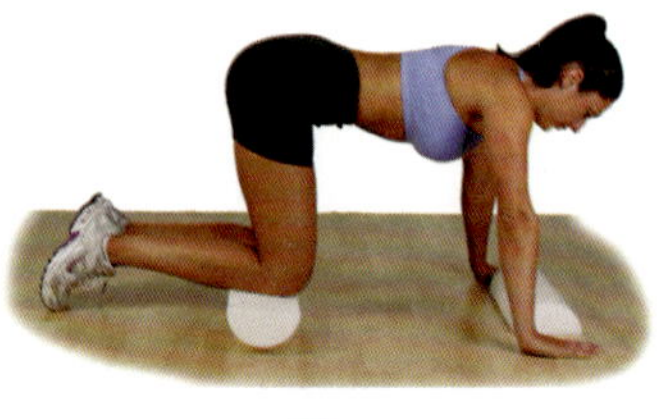

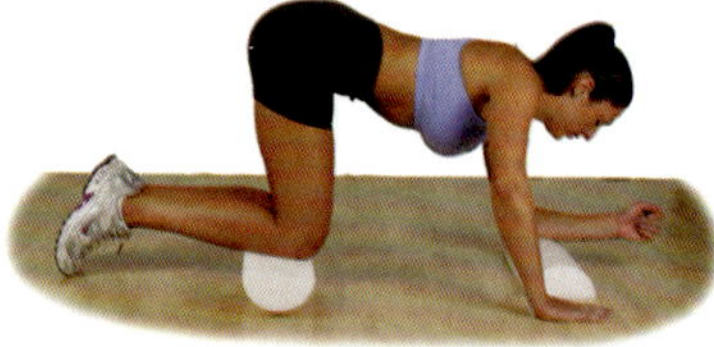

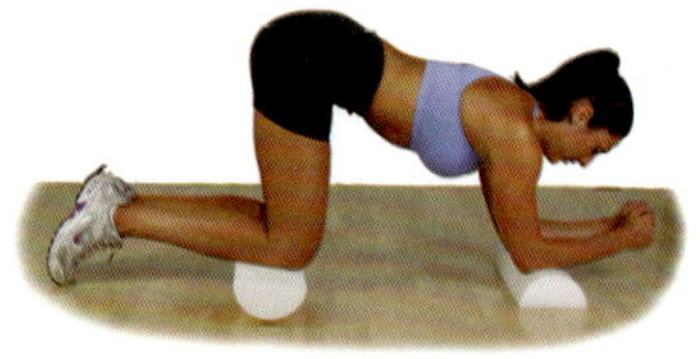

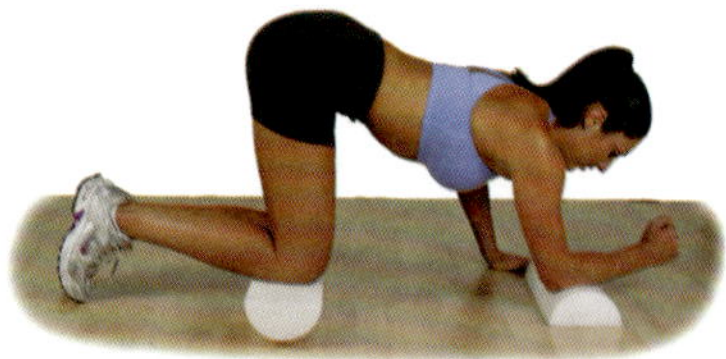

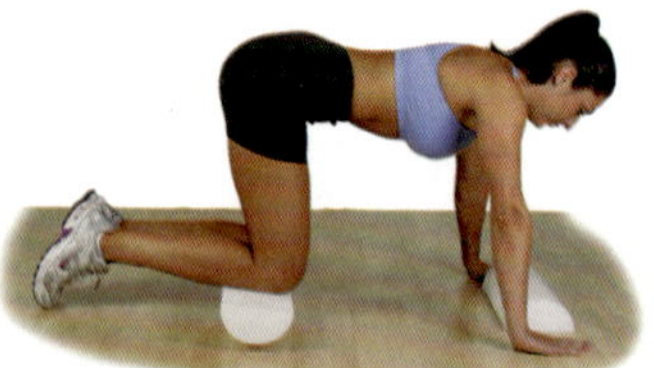

Progression:

1. Move your knees further back, away from your hands.
2. Then, instead of bending your elbows, keep them straight and walk your hands toward your knees to a six o'clock position (see photo).
3. Balance on your feet instead of your knees, and walk your hands to the six o'clock position, as in step 2 above.

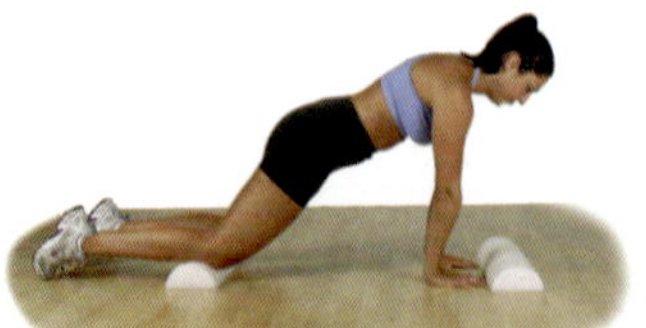

Hands at six o'clock position

Reach for the Stars

Muscles worked: deltoid, scapular retractors, erector spinae, spinal rotators, anatomical girdle, pelvis and hip stabilizers, hip extensors

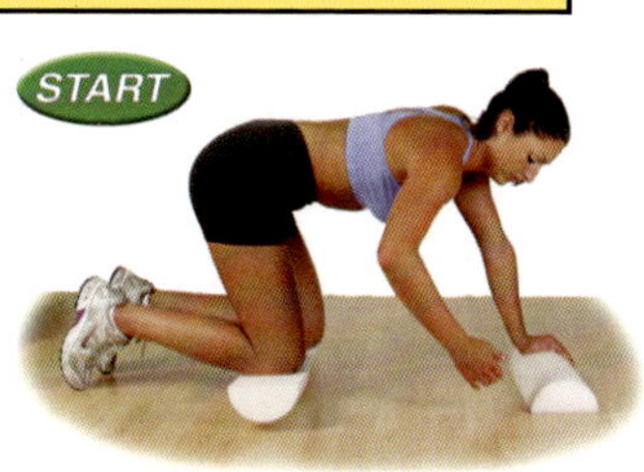

1. Kneel on a half roller.
2. Place your hands on a half or full roller laid crosswise in front of you.
3. Perform the Girdle Grip (pg. 8).
4. Transfer your weight to your left arm and raise your right arm off the roller.
5. Turning your torso to the right, reach up as high as you can while maintaining proper posture.
6. Allow your spine and head to naturally rotate and assist your reach for the ceiling.
7. Hold this position for 5 seconds.
8. Return to the starting position and sweep your right arm under your body, toward the left.
9. Hold this position for 5 seconds.
10. Repeat 5 times and switch sides.

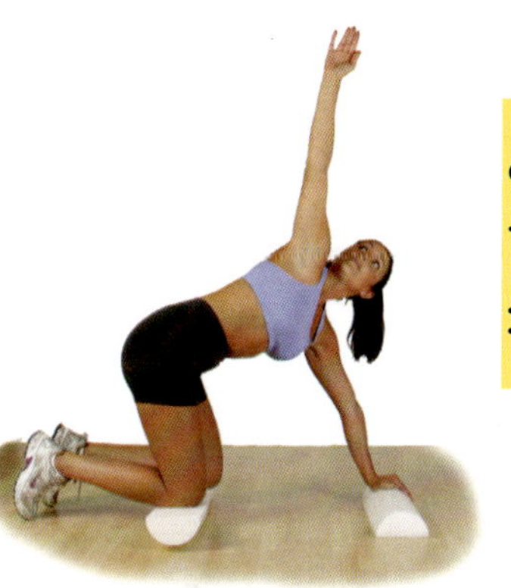

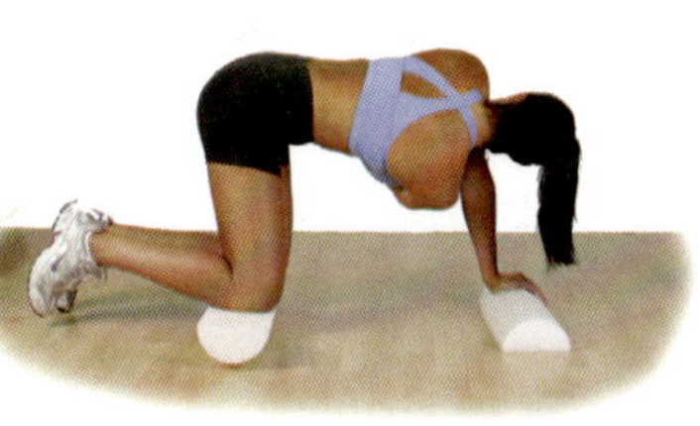

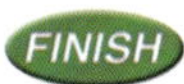

Note:

1. As you raise one arm to the ceiling, keep the supporting arm straight and maintain a strong Girdle Grip (pg. 8).
2. Do not sit back on your heels.
3. Remember to breathe throughout the exercise.

Progression:

1. Increase to 12 repetitions with 5-second holds in each position.
2. Hold a 1 to 3 pound dumbbell in your raised hand.
3. Move from your knees to your feet, and your hands to your elbows (still balanced on rollers), and perform the exercise in this more challenging position.

Kneeling Exercises

One Arm Dumbbell Raise

Muscles worked: deltoid, erector spinae, anatomical girdle, spine, pelvis and hip stabilizers

START

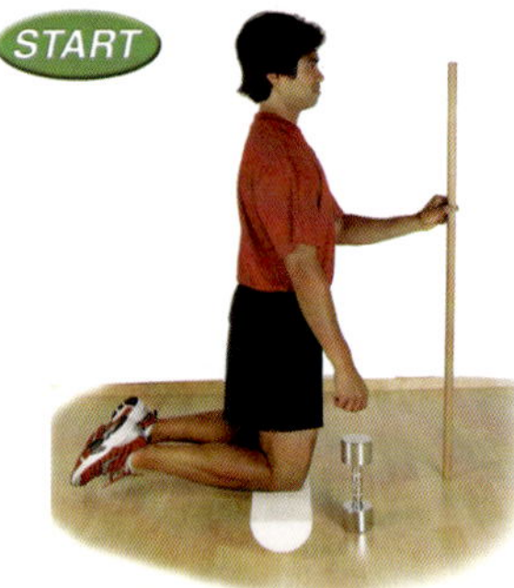

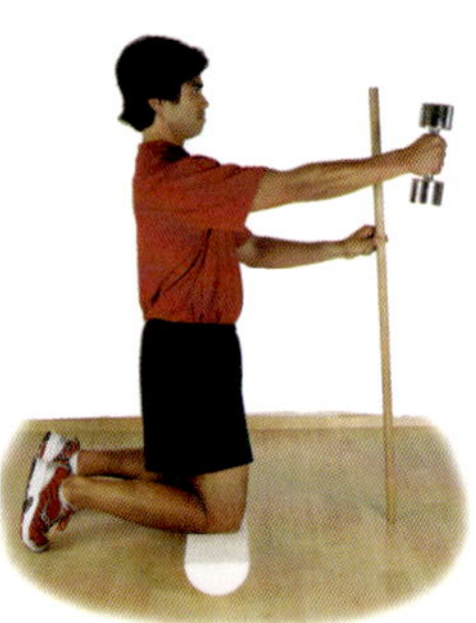

FINISH

Kneeling

1. Kneel on a half roller with your knees on the flat surface.
2. If needed, use a broomstick, held with thumb and forefinger only, to maintain your balance.
3. Perform the Girdle Grip (pg. 8). Imagine a broomstick against your spine.
4. Hold a dumbbell in your right hand and raise your arm straight out in front of you. Do not sit back on your heels.
5. Hold this position for 5 seconds. Remember to breathe throughout the exercise.
6. Repeat 5 times and switch sides.

Progression:

1. Increase to 12 repetitions with 5-second holds.
2. Use a full roller (with or without the stick).

Variation:

Try holding the dumbbell at different angles.

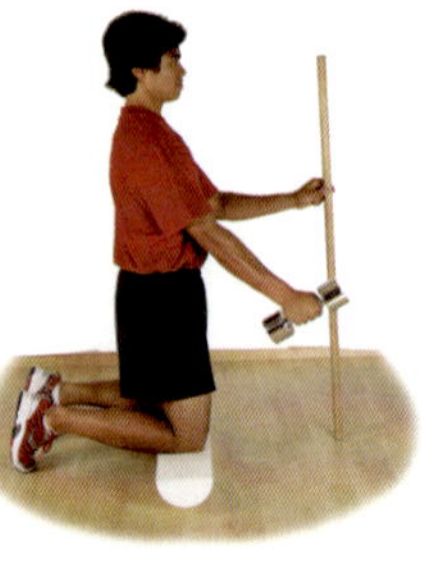

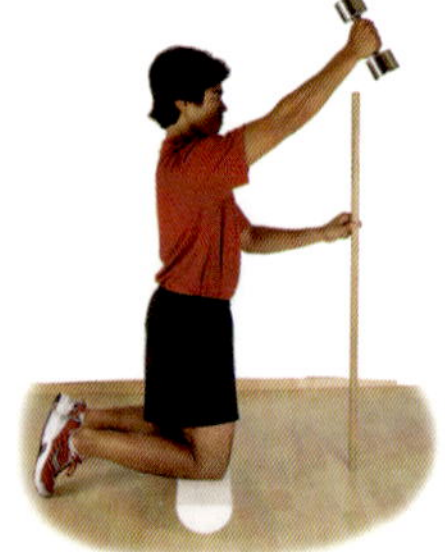

Tubing Samurai Twist

Muscles worked: spinal rotators, deltoid, external rotator cuff, chest, erector spinae, anatomical girdle, spine, pelvis and hip stabilizers

START

1. Anchor an exercise stretch tube at mid-waist level (when kneeling, so you can pull it evenly across your body).
2. Kneel on a half roller with your knees on the flat surface (round side down).
3. Grip the tube handle with both hands.
4. Perform the Girdle Grip (pg. 8). Imagine a broomstick against your spine.
5. With your arms straight, stretch the tube.
6. Begin with your shoulders and spine rotated toward the anchor point.
7. Then pull the tubing around to your left.
8. Hold this position for 5 seconds.
9. Repeat 5 times and switch sides.

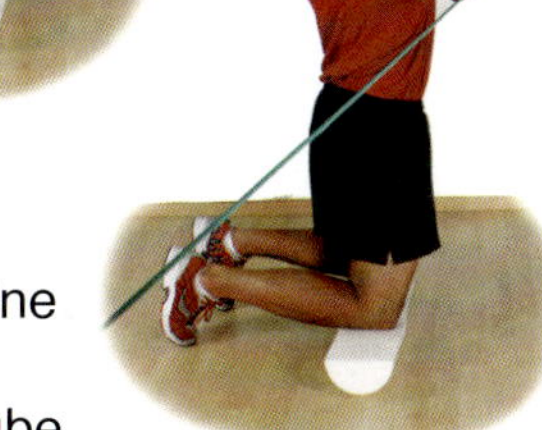

FINISH

Progression:
1. Increase to 12 repetitions with 5-second holds.
2. Use a full roller.

Variation:
Anchor the tubing very low and pull the tubing from low to high.

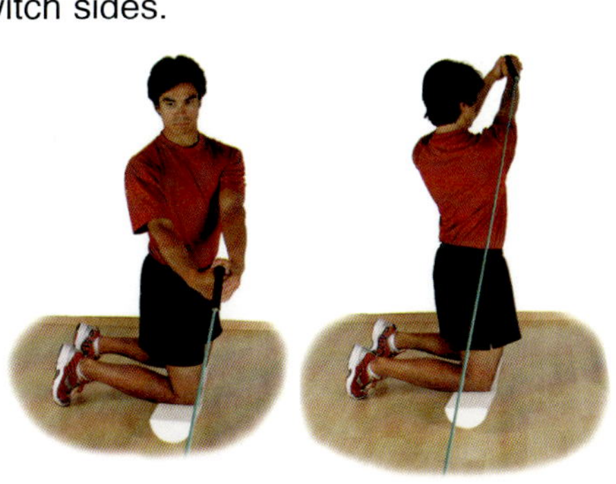

Tubing Stride Single Arm

Muscles worked: spinal rotators, deltoid, chest, erector spinae, anatomical girdle, spine, pelvis and hip stabilizers

1. Anchor an exercise stretch tube at mid-waist level (when kneeling, so you can pull it evenly across your body).
2. Kneel on a half roller with your right knee, and place your left foot in front of you on another roller (for more stability put your foot on the floor).
3. Grip the tube handle with your left hand. Start with the tubing taut.
4. Perform the Girdle Grip (pg. 8). Imagine a broomstick against your spine.
5. Start with your torso rotated toward the anchor point, your arm straight, your shoulders down, and your arm in line with the tubing.
6. Slowly pull the tubing across your body from left to right.
7. Hold this position for 5 seconds.
8. Repeat 5 times and switch sides.

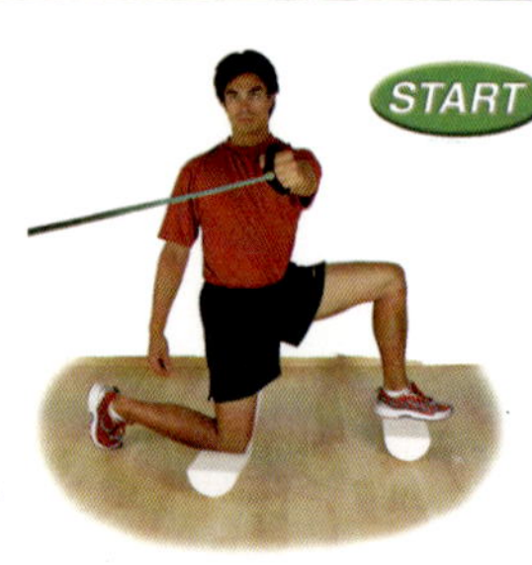

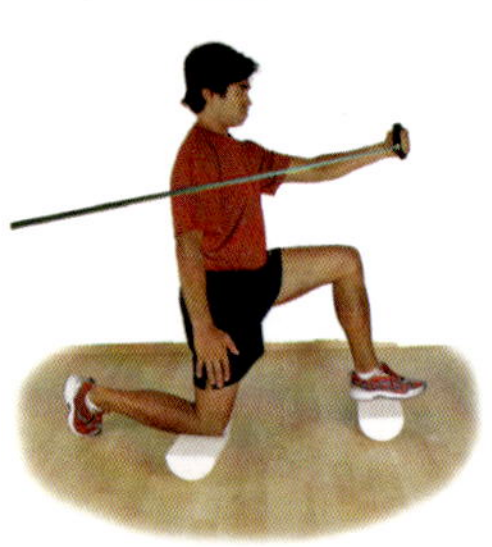

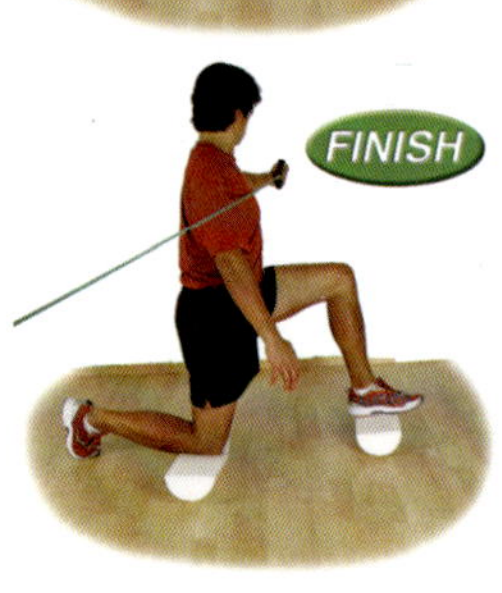

Progression:
1. Increase to 12 repetitions with 5-second holds.
2. Use a full roller under one or both legs.

Variation: Vary the tubing's anchor height and pull the tubing from low to high, and high to low.

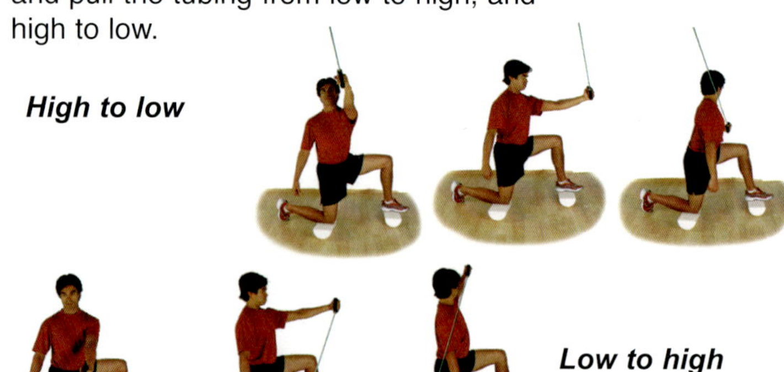

Tubing Stride Double Arm

Muscles worked: spinal rotators, deltoid, chest, erector spinae, anatomical girdle, spine, pelvis and hip stabilizers

1. Anchor an exercise stretch tube at mid waist level (when kneeling, so you can pull it evenly across your body).
2. Kneel on a half roller with your right knee, and place your left foot in front of you on another roller (for more stability put your foot on the floor).
3. Grip the tube handle with both hands. Start with the tubing taut.
4. Perform the Girdle Grip (pg. 8). Imagine a broomstick against your spine.
5. Start with your torso rotated toward the anchor point, your arm straight, your shoulders down, and your arm in line with the tubing.
6. Slowly pull the tubing across your body from left to right.
7. Hold this position for 5 seconds.
8. Repeat 5 times and switch sides.

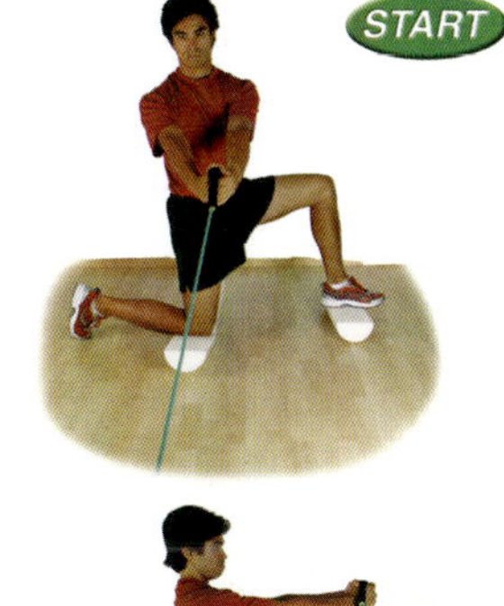

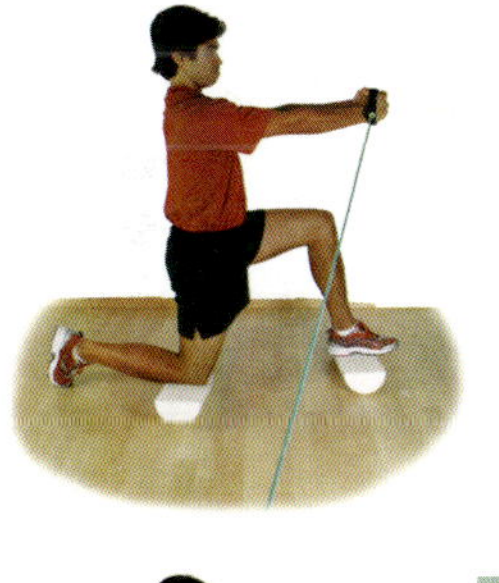

FINISH

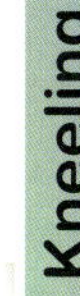

Progression:

1. Increase to 12 repetitions with 5-second holds.
2. Use a full roller under one or both legs.

Variation: Vary the tubing's anchor height and pull the tubing from low to high, and high to low.

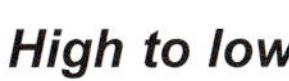

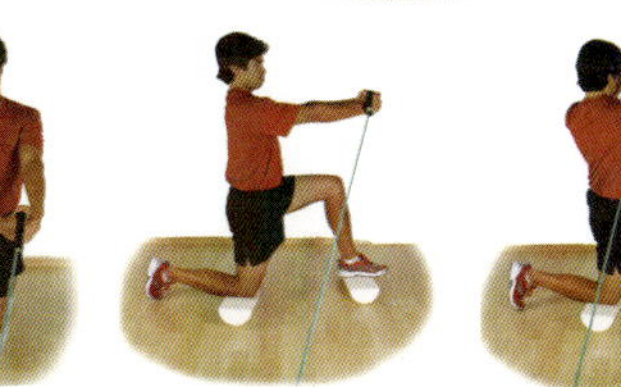

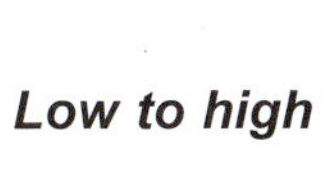

Lying Face Up EXERCISES

Ramping

Muscles worked: erector spinae, pelvis and hip stabilizers, hip extensors **Variation:** plus adductors

1. Lay on your back with your knees bent.
2. Place your feet hip-width apart on a half roller.
3. Perform the Girdle Grip (pg. 8). For balance, place your arms slightly to the side.
4. Raise your pelvis off the floor until your body is straight like a ramp.
5. Hold this position for 5 seconds.
6. Lower your buttocks – but stop just before you reach the floor.
7. Repeat 5 times.

Progression:

1. Increase to 12 repetitions with 5-second holds in the Ramp position.
2. Remove your arms from the floor and cross them over your chest.
3. Lay on a half roller running lengthwise from your head to your buttocks.

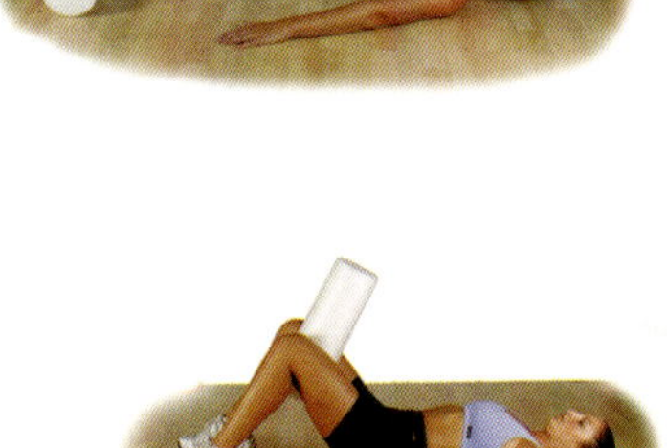

Variations:

1. Squeeze a roller between your knees while “ramping up”.
2. Wrap an exercise tube around your knees and push your legs out while ramping up.

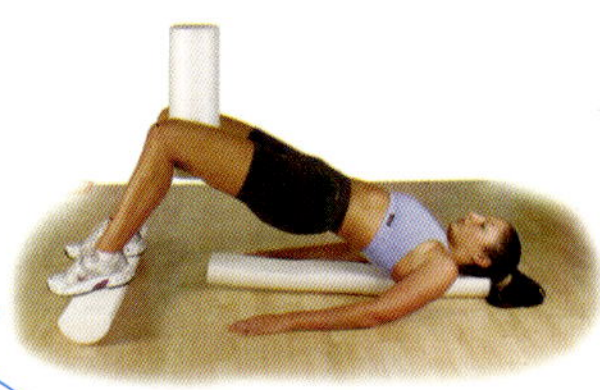

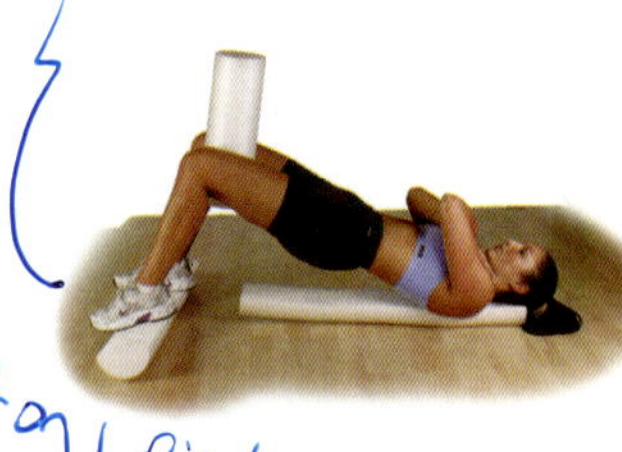

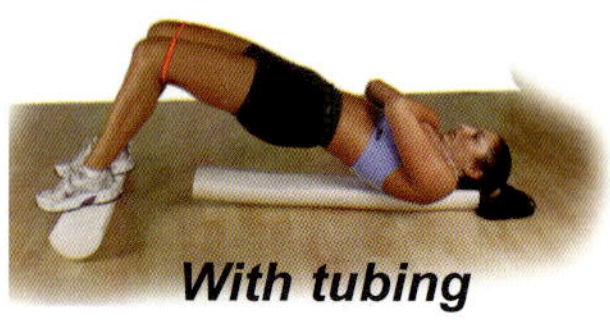

With tubing

Ramp and Track

Muscles worked: neck rotators, chest, erector spinae, pelvis and hip stabilizers, hip extensors

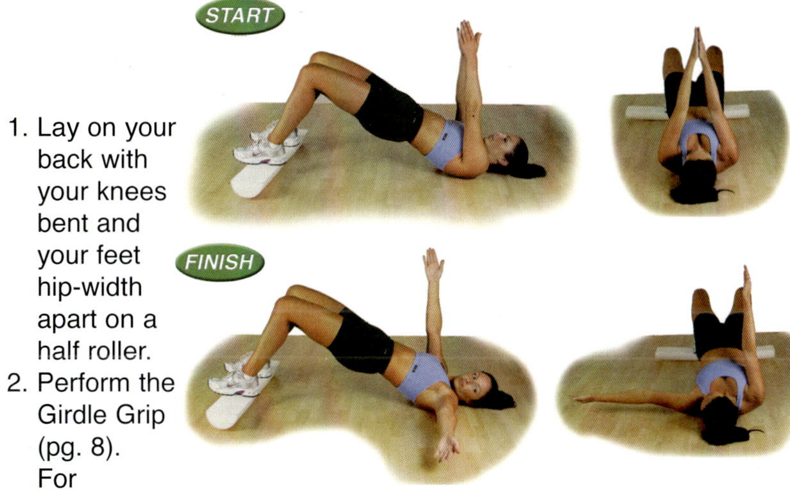

1. Lay on your back with your knees bent and your feet hip-width apart on a half roller.
2. Perform the Girdle Grip (pg. 8). For balance, place your arms slightly to the side.
3. Raise your arms straight up toward the ceiling and press your palms together.
4. Raise your pelvis off the floor until your body is straight like a ramp.
5. Lower your left arm toward the floor and track the movement with your eyes – turn your head to follow your arm. All movements should be slow and controlled.
6. Stop just before you reach the floor and hold for 5 seconds.
7. Raise your arm to point at the ceiling again.
8. Lower your buttocks – but stop just before you reach the floor.
9. Repeat 3 times and switch sides.

Progression:

1. Increase to 6 repetitions with 5-second holds for each arm.
2. Hold a 1 to 5 pound dumbbell in the arm you lower toward the floor.
3. Ramp-up on the leg opposite to the arm you are lowering. For example, balance on your right leg while you lower your left arm.

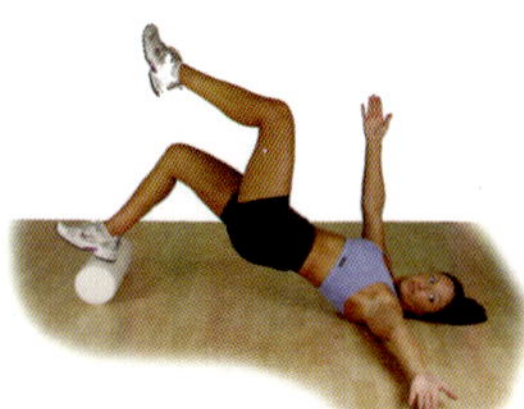

Advanced

Ramp & Scissor

Muscles worked: hamstrings, calves, erector spinae, pelvis and hip stabilizers, hip extensors

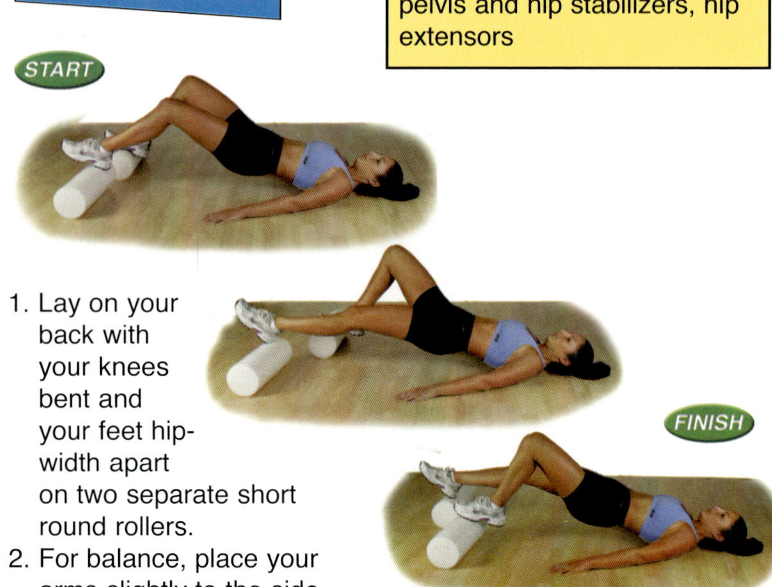

1. Lay on your back with your knees bent and your feet hip-width apart on two separate short round rollers.
2. For balance, place your arms slightly to the side.
3. Perform the Girdle Grip (pg. 8).
4. Raise your pelvis off the floor until your body is straight like a ramp.
5. Maintaining balance on the rollers, roll your left foot away and your right foot toward you.
6. Pause when your right leg is extended and your left foot is close to your buttocks. Hold for 5 seconds.
7. Then reverse the direction of the rollers so your left foot is close to your buttocks and your right leg is extended.
8. Hold for another 5 seconds.
9. Return your feet to the starting position.
10. Lower your buttocks – but stop just before you reach the floor.
11. Repeat 3 times.

Progression:

1. Increase to 6 repetitions with 5-second holds.
2. Remove your arms from the floor and cross them over your chest.

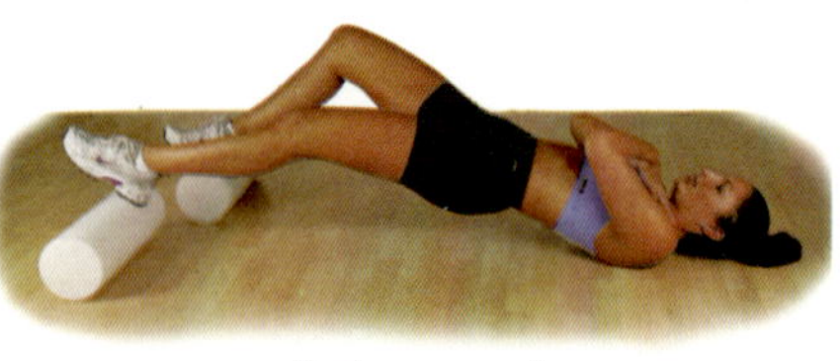

Advanced

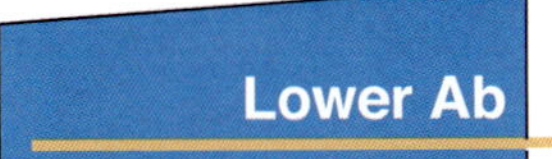

Lower Ab

Muscles worked: erector spinae, lower abdominals, pelvis and hip stabilizers

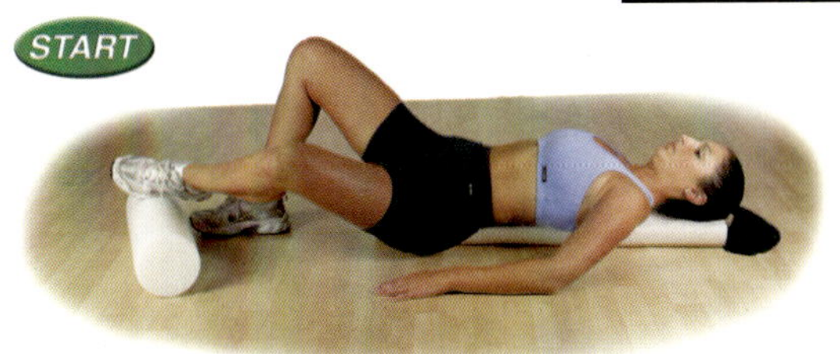

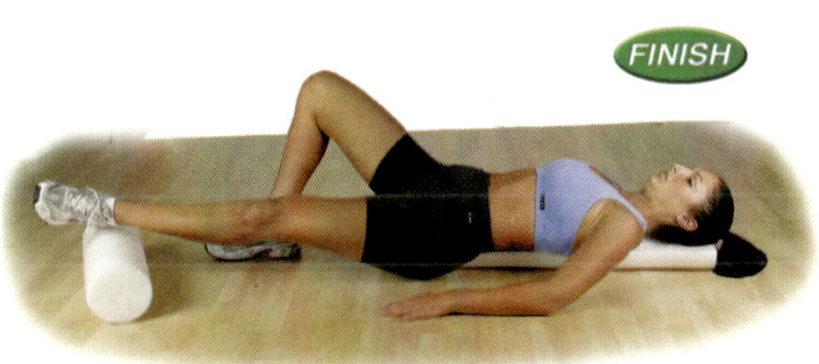

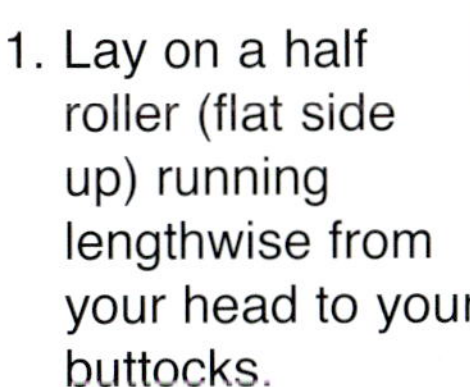

1. Lay on a half roller (flat side up) running lengthwise from your head to your buttocks.
2. Bend your knees and place your feet hip-width apart.
3. Place the toes of your left foot on a short roller. Leave your right foot flat on the floor.
4. For balance, place your arms slightly to the side.
5. Perform the Girdle Grip (pg. 8). Imagine a broomstick against your spine.
6. Start by dropping your left knee to the left, and roll your left foot away from you.
7. Stop at a comfortable extension and hold for 5 seconds.
8. Return to the starting position.
9. Repeat 5 times and then switch sides.

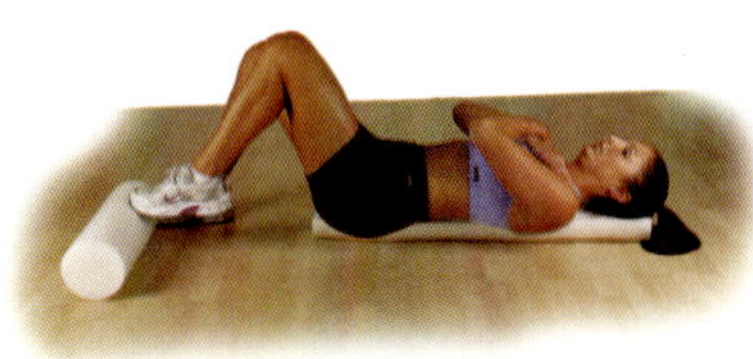

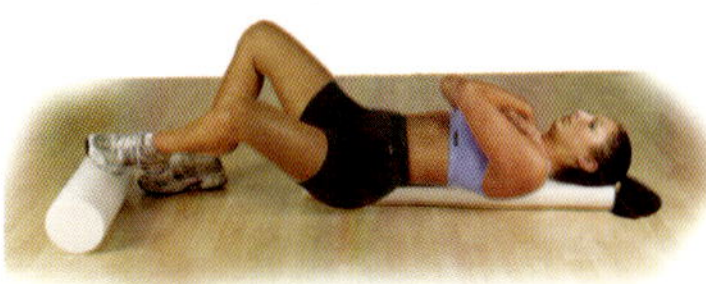

Advanced

Progression:

1. Increase to 12 repetitions with 5-second holds.
2. Remove your arms from the floor and cross them over your chest.

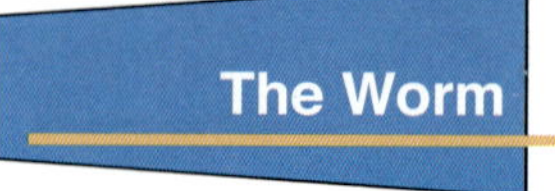

Muscles worked: erector spinae, quadratus lumborum, obliques (lateral fibers), scapular depressors

START

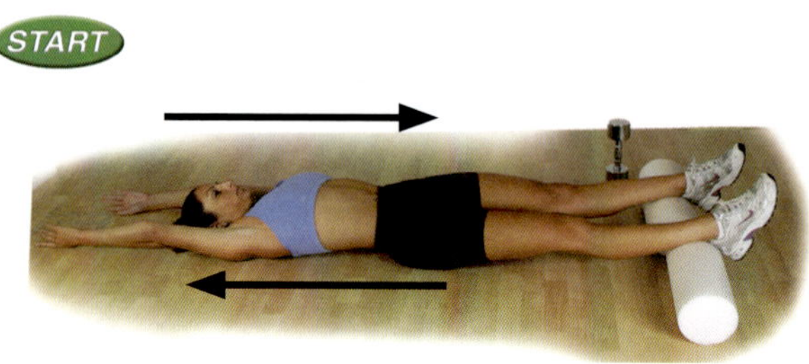

FINISH

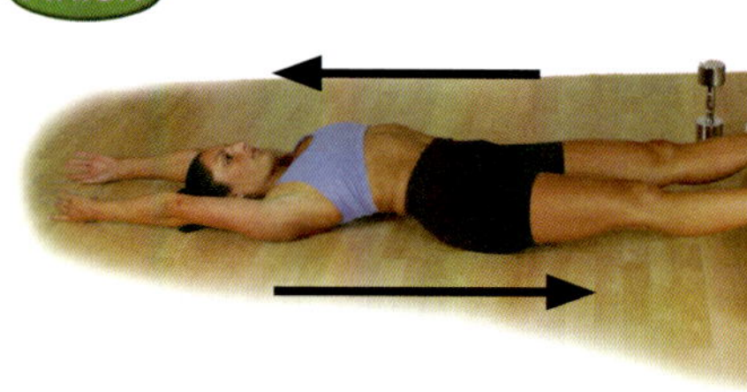

1. Lay on your back with your legs straight.
2. Place your feet hip-width apart on two separate short rollers.
3. Lay your arms on the floor above your head.
4. Perform the Girdle Grip (pg. 8).
5. Reach your left arm along the floor, as far away from your head as possible
6. At the same time, slide the right hip (opposite to your arm) up toward your right armpit.
7. Hold for 1 second and then switch sides.
8. Don't arch or flatten your lower back – maintain neutral alignment.
9. Repeat this "worm" movement for 10 seconds.

Note: This is a fantastic exercise to combat lower back pain.

Progression: Increase your Worm wiggle time to 60 seconds.

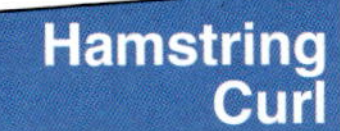

Hamstring Curl

Muscles worked: hamstrings, gastrocnemius, erector spinae, pelvis and hip stabilizers, hip extensors

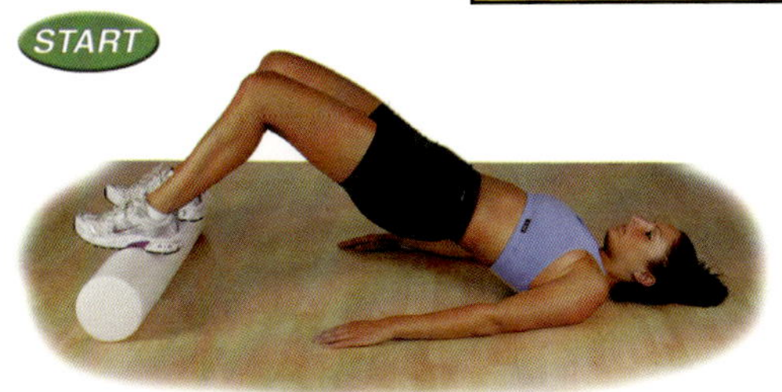

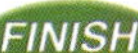

1. Lay on your back with your knees bent.
2. Place your feet hip-width apart on a long full roller.
3. For balance, place your arms slightly to the side.
4. Perform the Girdle Grip (pg. 8).
5. Raise your pelvis off the floor until your body is straight like a ramp.
6. Roll both feet away from you.
7. Stop at a comfortable extension and hold for 5 seconds.
8. Return to the starting position.
9. Repeat 5 times.

Note: Do not drop your buttocks at any stage during this exercise.

Progression:

1. Increase to 12 repetitions with 5-second holds.
2. Remove your arms from the floor and cross them over your chest.
3. During your 5-second hold in the extended position, place your hands on your pelvis and tilt your pelvis to the left and then the right.

Lying Sideways EXERCISES

Inner Thigh Side Ramp

Muscles worked: hip adductors of the top leg, lateral obliques, spinal and shoulder stabilizers of the bottom arm

1. Place your right elbow on a half roller, perpendicular to the roller.
2. Lay on your side with your knees bent and together.
3. Perform the Girdle Grip (pg. 8). Imagine a broomstick against your spine.
4. Raise your pelvis sideways off the floor until the center of your hips, belly button, chest, neck and head are all aligned.

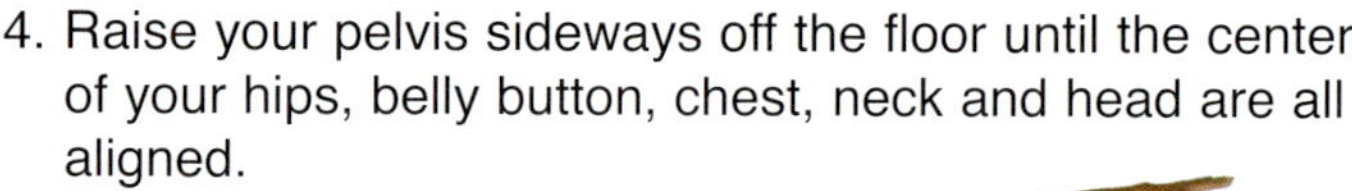

5. Cross your lower leg behind your upper leg.
6. Hold this position for 5 seconds.
7. Lower your pelvis – but stop just before you reach the floor.
8. Repeat 5 times and switch sides.

Progression:

1. Increase your hold time to 60 seconds but only repeat the exercise twice.
2. With your free arm, perform small 3-inch arm movements, such as circles and up/down movements.
3. Hold a 1 to 5 pound dumbbell as you perform the arm movements.

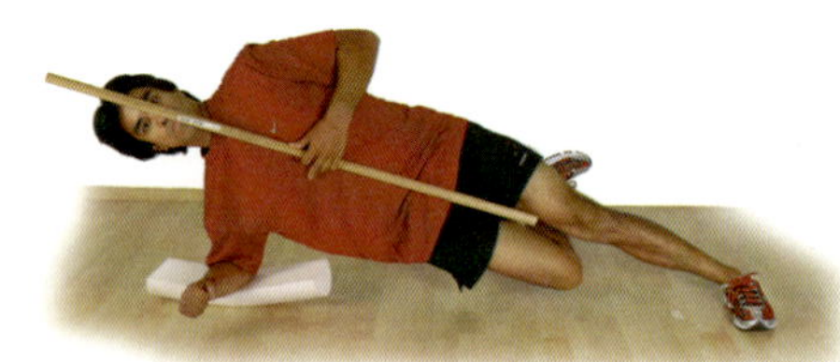

To learn neutral spinal alignment, use your left hand to hold a stick against your chest, lengthwise along your body. Have someone check your alignment (or look in a mirror).

Variation: Place your top knee (left leg) on a short roller. Position the roller below the knee. The full roller is merely a means for relieving body weight on the working muscles.

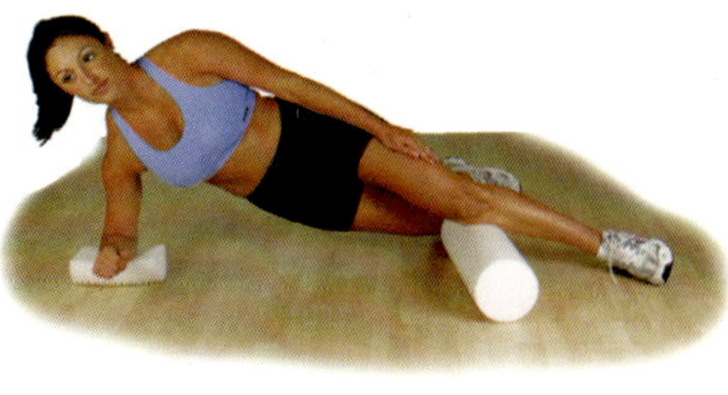

Note:
1. The foot and inner thigh of your top leg will provide most of your leverage.

Progression:
1. Increase your hold time to 60 seconds but only repeat the exercise twice.
2. Remove the full roller from under your knee and straighten the leg.

Elbow Position

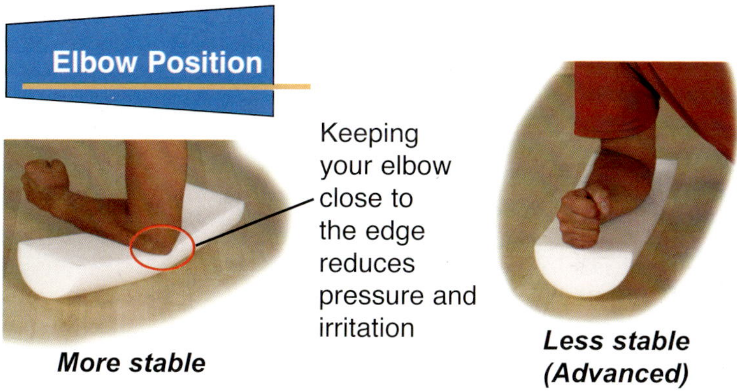

More stable

Less stable (Advanced)

1. In this and the following exercises, you should take care when placing your elbow on the half roller.
2. To avoid irritating the bursa of the elbow, ensure your elbow is as close as possible to the edge of the half roller.
3. Place as much weight on the forearm as is comfortable. However, some weight must remain on the elbow to maintain proper technique.

Note: Those with IT Band Syndrome should consult a physical therapist before performing Side Ramp Novice and Side Ramp Advanced. See pages 59 to 60 for massage of the IT Band.

Outer Thigh Side Ramp

Muscles worked: abductors of the bottom hip, lateral obliques, spinal and shoulder stabilizers

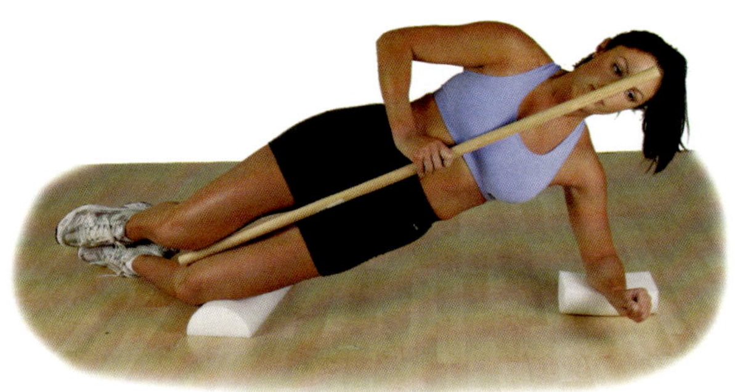

1. Place your right elbow on a half roller, perpendicular to the roller (see Elbow Position pg. 49).
2. Place your bottom right leg behind you, and your top left leg slightly in front of you.
3. Anchor your top leg by pressing the sole of your left foot into the floor.
4. Perform the Girdle Grip (pg. 8). Imagine a broomstick against your spine.
5. Raise your pelvis off the floor until your hips, belly button, chest, neck and head are all aligned.
6. Hold this position for 5 seconds and then slowly lower your pelvis, - but stop just before you reach the floor.
7. Repeat 5 times and switch sides.

Note: Don't sag in the shoulder area. Push your shoulder out to prevent sagging.

MYOFACIAL RELEASE

The term "myofascial release" is actually self explanatory. "Myo" means muscle; "fascia" is the sheet of tissue connecting the muscles; and "release" refers to separating the adhesions between the fascia and the muscles.

You can think of fascia as a seamless unit of cellophane wrapped around and through every muscle and tissue in your body. In fact you can see it for yourself. If you ever pull the fat and skin off a chicken, look for the transparent, cellophane-like wrapping around the chicken's muscle. That's fascia.

This tough cellophane-like layer is supposed to glide along and against other tissue such as fat, muscles, nerves and other fascia. However due to injury, or lack of movement, fascia can adhere or stick to the underside of tissue such as skin, blood vessels and nerves. Eventually, these adhesions restrict blood circulation, nerve transmission and tissue health. Adhesions also impact movement, sleep and quality of daily living – creating chronic back, neck, hip and leg pain.

The myofascial unit can be compared to a large, body-wide sweater, where fascia is the yarn. If yarn in one part of the sweater is damaged or pulled out of shape (fascial adhesions) then the tugging or imbalance will affect other parts of the body.

Myofascial release targets these adhesions to return health and balance to your body.

Test Myofascial Release for Yourself

Try the following to get a feel for myofascial release:

1. Sit in a chair and roll a short roller up and down one thigh.
2. Use the roller to search for tender spots in the thigh muscles.
3. Once you find a tender spot – called a "pain spot" – firmly roll over it for about 90 seconds.
4. Generally the tender spot feels better, which is known as a "release" of pain or tension.
5. Then search for another tender spot.

Let Pain be Your Guide

It is important to realize that with myofascial release, some pain is normal. The guidelines of the Soreness Test (pg. 7) do not apply here.

However, determining the right level of pain is a personal

process of trial and error. Those with a "go-for-it" attitude to exercise tend to like the greater-pain faster-release approach. Others prefer a gentler, less-pain more-comfort method. In choosing your preferred approach, you will need to pay careful attention to your body's feedback during and after the massage.

During the Massage

While practicing myofascial release it is normal to experience the following sensations in and around the tender spot you are massaging:

- An increase in pain
- A tingling sensation
- A burning feeling

After the Massage

Normal results in the massaged body area include:

- Warmth
- Redness
- Improved circulation
- Decreased pain

Poor results include:

- Bruising
- Loss of sensation
- Increased sensitivity to touch
- Decreased limb function
- Increased pain

If you experience any of the poor results, you should:

- Stop the massage
- Seek professional guidance

Note: Those with limb circulatory problems and chronic pain diseases (such as fibromyalgia) should consult an appropriate health care professional before using foam rollers.

Maximizing the Benefits

To get the most out of your myofascial release session, follow this post-massage process:

- Place the massaged muscle in a relaxed position – do not contract the muscle.
- Gently stretch the muscle.
- Apply ice (frozen in a paper cup) in a gentle, stroking manner in the direction of the muscle.
- Perform 3 strokes along the area at 4 inches per second, then gently stretch again.
- Heat the area with a warm – not hot – heat pad.
- Repeat 2 to 3 times.

Back Release

Purpose: Massages back muscles and improves spine and rib cage range of motion.

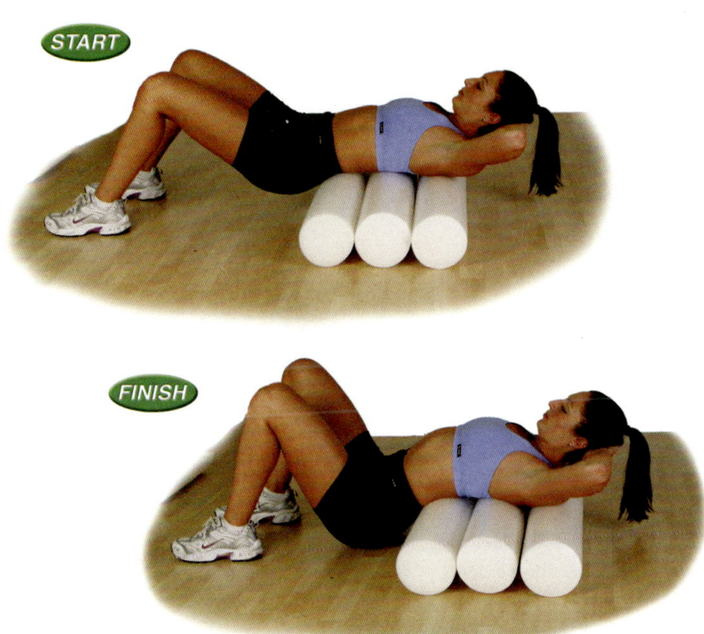

1. Place 1 to 3 rollers together on the floor – more rollers means more support and massage.
2. Lay on your back with the roller(s) under your shoulders and spine.
3. Bend your knees and keep your feet flat on the floor.
4. Perform the Girdle Grip (pg. 8).
5. Place your hands behind your head for additional support.
6. Stabilize your neck muscles to maintain a neutral neck/ head alignment.
7. Gently roll back and forth, massaging your back, feeling for muscle "pain spots".
8. Once you find a tender spot, roll over it firmly until you feel the tension release.
9. Then feel for another pain spot.

Variation:

Perform the exercise standing and place the roller(s) against a wall, instead of the floor.

Quad Release

Purpose: Massages quadriceps.

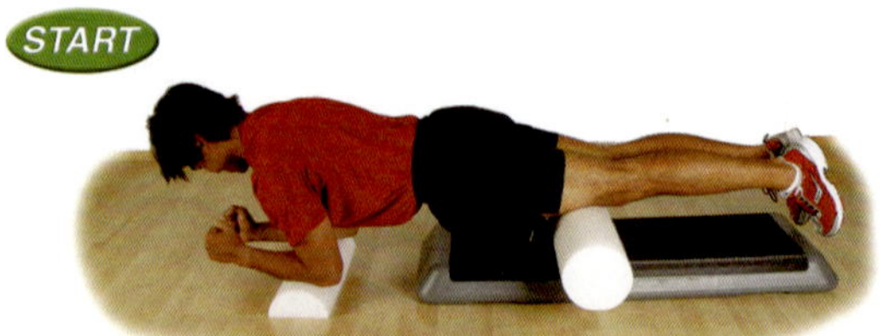

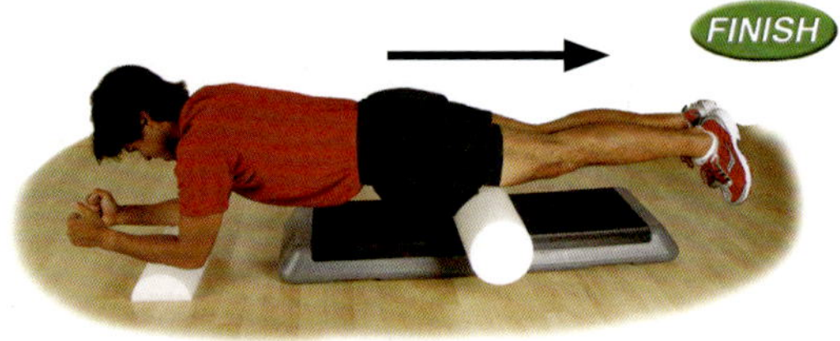

Elevated surface

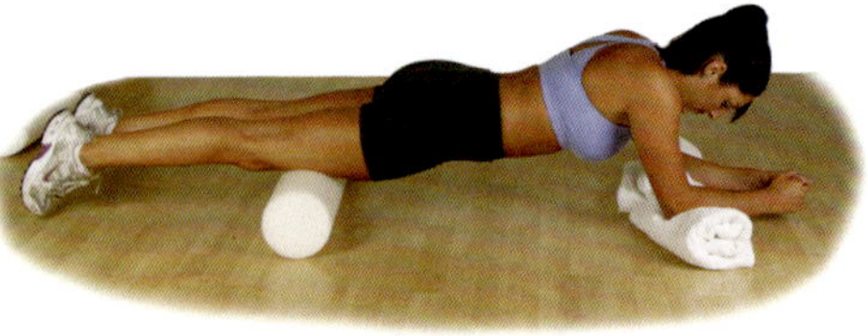

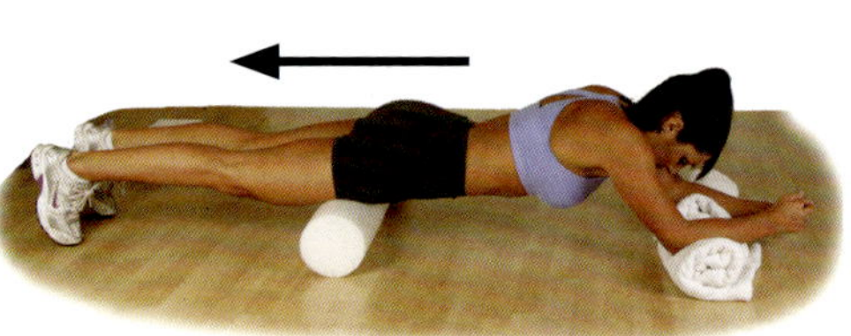

Flat surface

1. Place a full roller on an elevated flat surface, or on the floor.
2. Lay face down with the roller positioned against your thighs, just above your knees.
3. Place your forearms on a half roller or towel, for upper body support.
4. Perform the Girdle Grip (pg. 8).
5. Stabilize your neck muscles to maintain a neutral neck/ head alignment – look at the floor.
6. Gently roll back and forth, feeling for pain spots.
7. Once you find a tender spot, roll over it firmly until you feel the tension release.
8. Then feel for another pain spot.

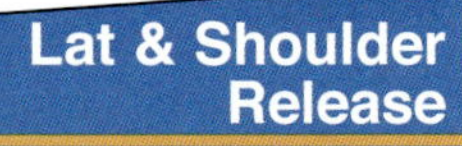

Lat & Shoulder Release

Purpose: Massages posterior deltoid, teres major, latissimus dorsi, and triceps.

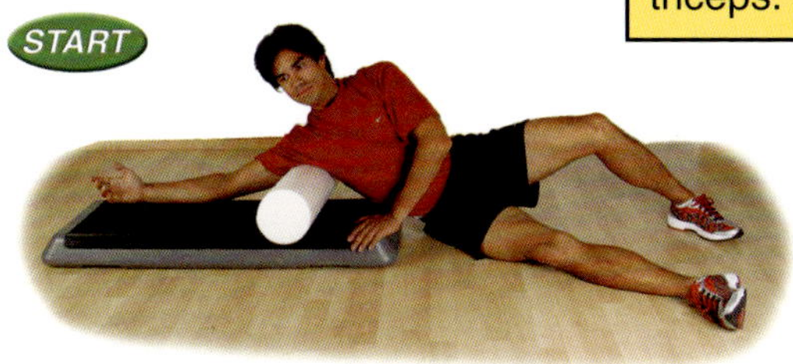

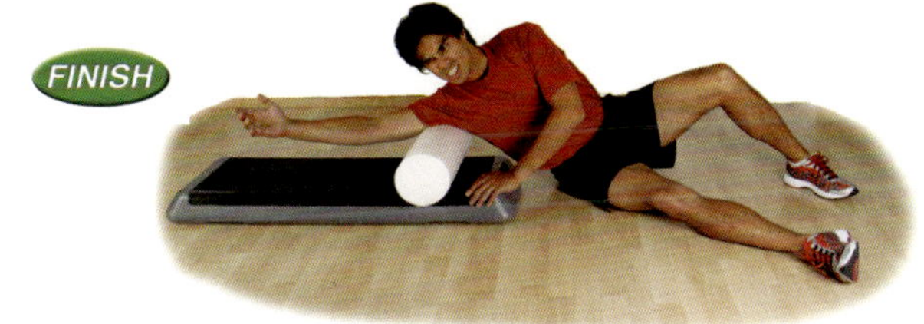

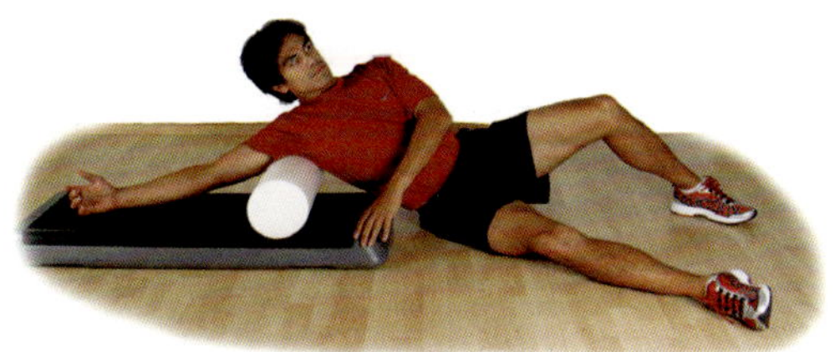

Lean back

1. Place a full roller on an elevated flat surface, or on the floor.
2. Lay on your side with the roller under your armpit.
3. Straighten your bottom leg and extend it slightly in front of you.
4. Bend your top leg and place your foot flat on the floor behind you for leverage (see photo).
5. Perform the Girdle Grip (pg. 8).
6. Straighten your bottom arm, and support yourself with your top arm.
7. Stabilize your neck muscles to maintain a neutral neck/head alignment – look forward.
8. Gently roll back and forth, feeling for pain spots.
9. Once you find a tender spot, roll over it firmly until you feel the tension release.
10. Then feel for another pain spot. Switch sides

Variation:
Lean back to increase the massage area.

T-Spine Release

Purpose: Massages erector spinae and scapular retractors.

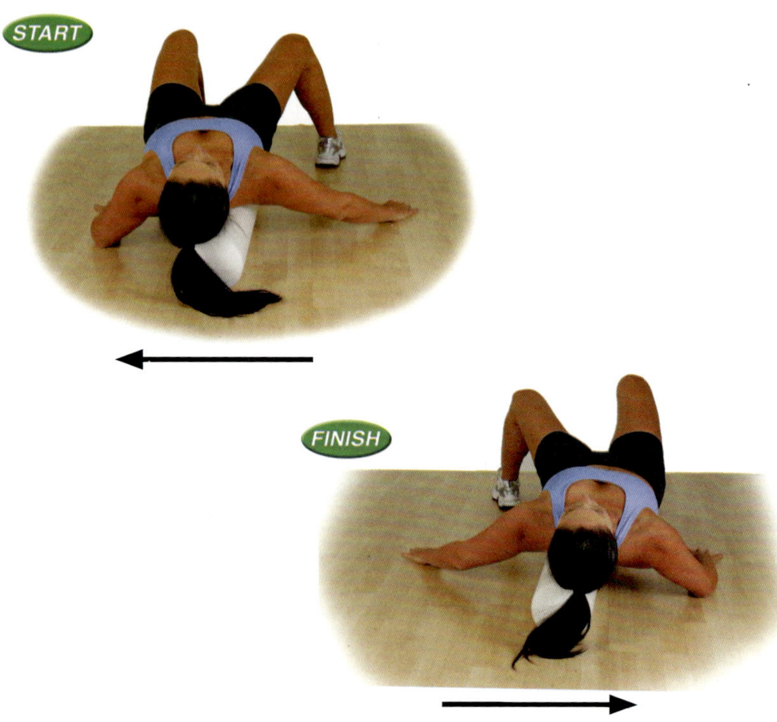

1. Place a long full roller on the floor.
2. Lay on your back so the roller runs lengthwise from your pelvis, up your spine, to your head.
3. Place your hands by your sides on the floor, for support.
4. Bend your knees and place your feet flat on the floor for leverage.
5. Perform the Girdle Grip (pg. 8).
6. Gently roll from side to side, feeling for pain spots.
7. Once you find a tender spot, roll over it firmly until you feel the tension release.
8. Then feel for another pain spot.

Variation:
Place the roller(s) against a wall, instead of the floor (not shown).

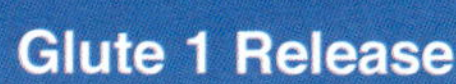

Glute 1 Release

Purpose: Massages gluteus maximus and origin of hamstrings.

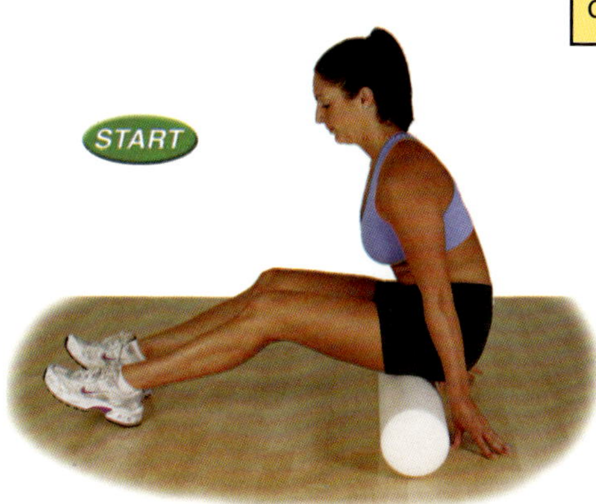

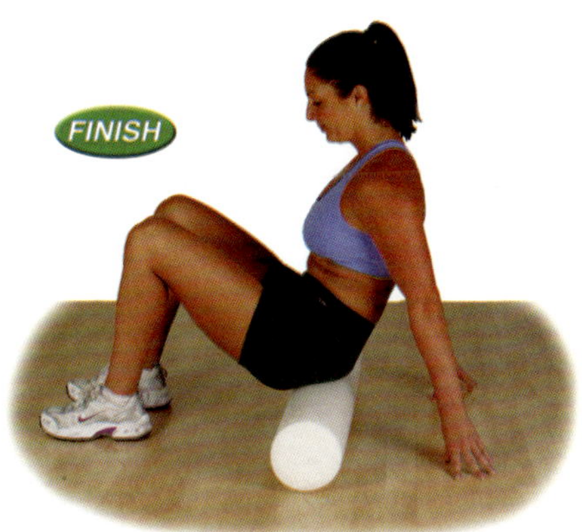

1. Place a full roller on the floor.
2. Sit with your buttocks hanging off the back of the roller.
3. Bend your knees and place your heels on the floor in front of you.
4. Place your hands by your sides on the floor, for support.
5. Perform the Girdle Grip (pg. 8).
6. Gently roll back and forth, massaging both buttocks, feeling for pain spots.
7. Once you find a tender spot, roll over it firmly until you feel the tension release.
8. Then feel for another pain spot.

Glute 2 Release

Purpose: Massages gluteus maximus and medius, posterior line of iliotibial band.

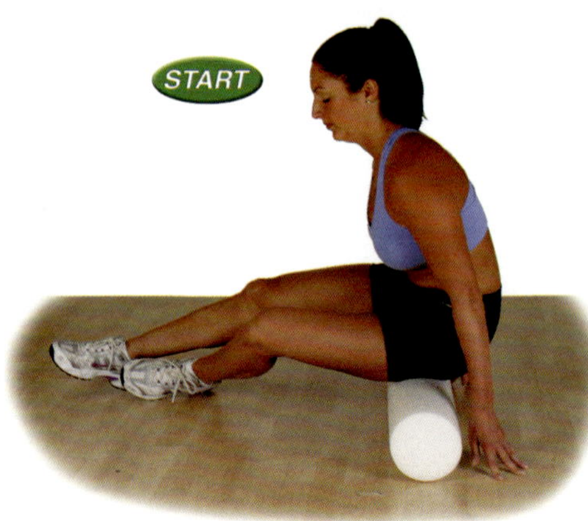

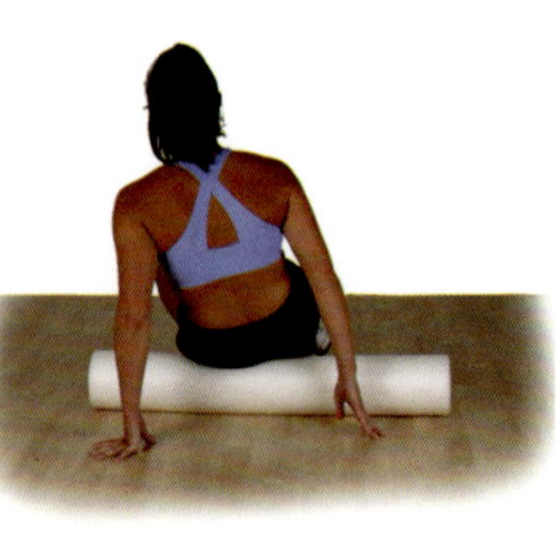

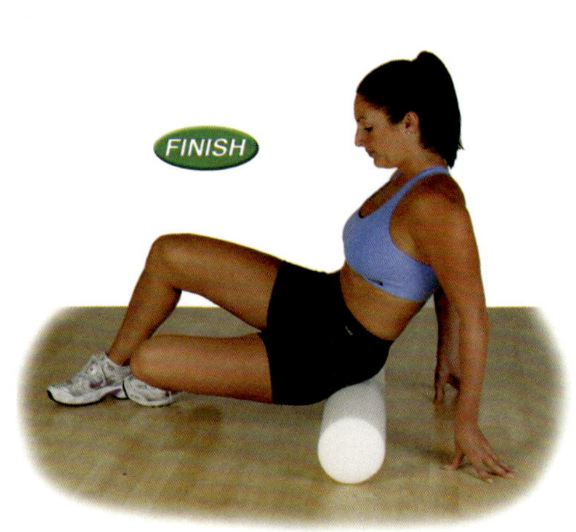

1. Place a full roller on the floor.
2. Sit on the roller with knees bent and your heels on the floor.
3. Place your hands by your sides on the floor, for support.
4. Lean left and drop your left knee to the side. This increases body weight on the left buttock (see photo).
5. Perform the Girdle Grip (pg. 8).
6. Gently roll back and forth, massaging your left buttock, feeling for pain spots.
7. Once you find a tender spot, roll over it firmly until you feel the tension release.
8. Then feel for another pain spot.
9. Switch sides.

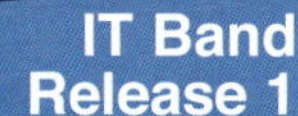

IT Band Release 1

Purpose: Massages anterior line of iliotibial band.

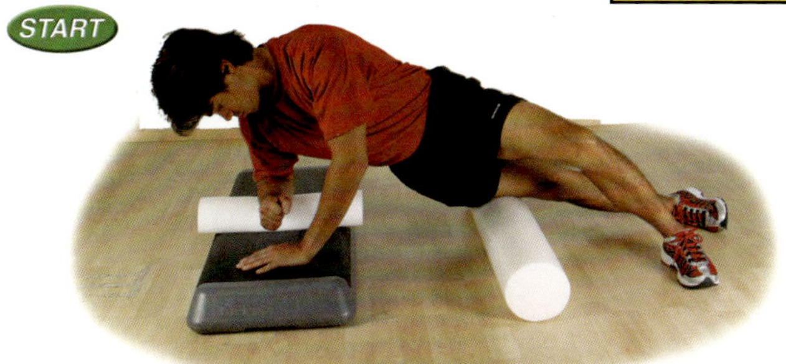

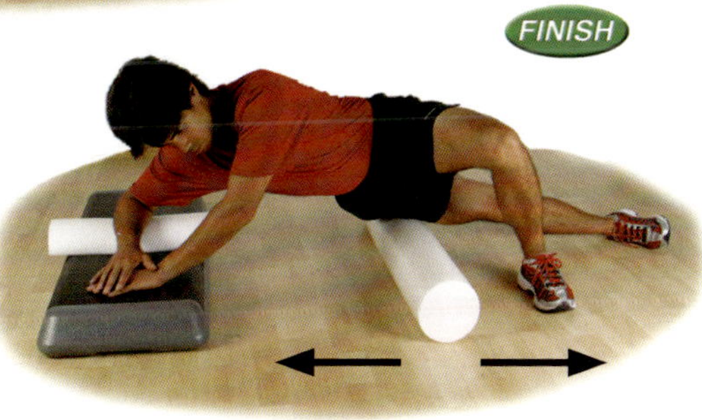

1. Place a half roller on an elevated flat surface, and a full roller on the floor.
2. Lay on your right side with your right elbow on the half roller.
3. Place your right leg, just above the knee, on the full roller.
4. Straighten your right leg and extend it slightly behind you.
5. Bend your left leg and place your foot flat on the floor slightly in front of you, for leverage.
6. Place your left arm in front of you on the elevated platform, for support.
7. Perform the Girdle Grip (pg. 8).
8. Stabilize your neck muscles to maintain a neutral neck/head alignment – look slightly downwards.
9. Gently roll back and forth, feeling for pain spots.
10. Once you find a tender spot, roll over it firmly until you feel the tension release.
11. Then feel for another pain spot.
12. Switch sides.

IT Band Release 2

Purpose: Massages posterior line of iliotibial band.

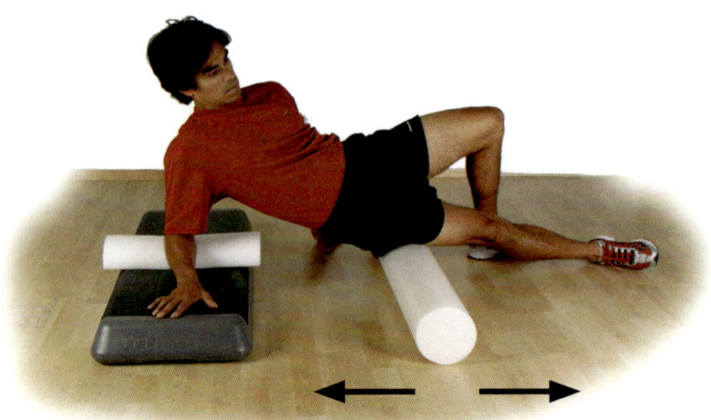

1. Place a half roller on an elevated flat surface, and a full roller on the floor.
2. Lay on your right side with your right elbow on the half roller.
3. Place your right leg, just above the knee, on the full roller.
4. Straighten your right leg and extend it slightly behind you.

Note: This exercise now differs from IT Band Release 1 (see pg. 58).

5. Bend your left leg and place your foot flat on the floor behind your right leg, for leverage.
6. Place your left arm behind you on the elevated platform for support (see photo).
7. Perform the Girdle Grip (pg. 8).
8. Stabilize your neck muscles to maintain a neutral neck/head alignment – look slightly downwards.
9. Gently roll back and forth, feeling for pain spots.
10. Once you find a tender spot, roll over it firmly until you feel the tension release.
11. Then feel for another pain spot.
12. Switch sides.

Variation:

Lean forward slightly to massage middle line of IT Band.

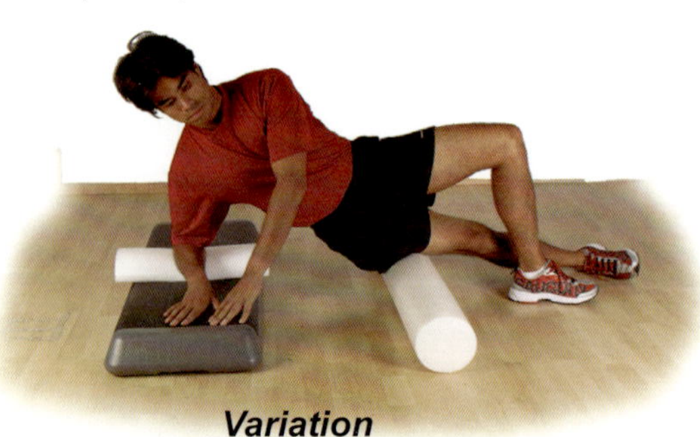

Variation

Inner Thigh Release

Purpose: Massages adductors.

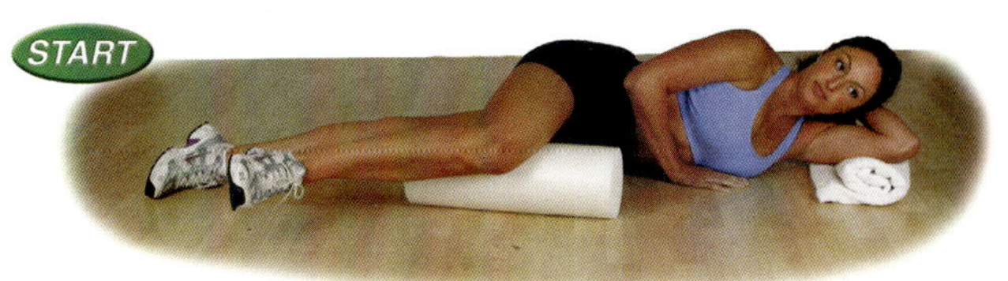

FINISH

1. Lay on your left side with your left arm folded under your head for support. You can use a towel (optional) for additional support.
2. Place a full roller beside you on the floor, or on an elevated flat surface.
3. Bend your top leg and place it on the roller, just above your knee.
4. Place your top arm on the floor in front of you, or on the elevated surface, for support.
5. Perform the Girdle Grip (pg. 8).
6. Gently roll your leg back and forth (by pushing your hips toward the roller), feeling for pain spots.
7. Once you find a tender spot, roll over it firmly until you feel the tension release.
8. Then feel for another pain spot.
9. Switch sides.

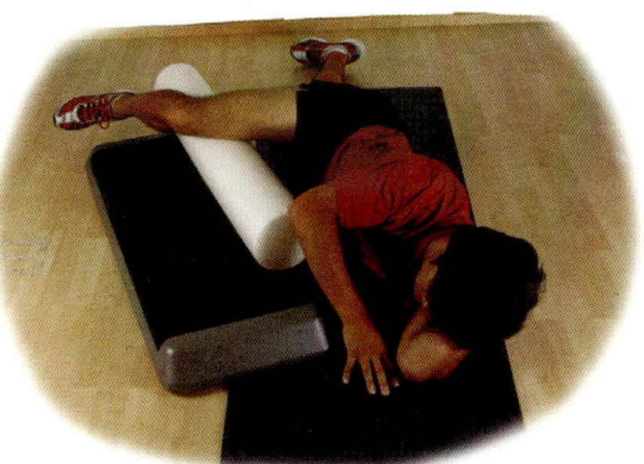

Variation 1

Variation 1:
Drop your top foot.

Variation 2:
Lift your top foot.

Both variations massage the inner thigh.

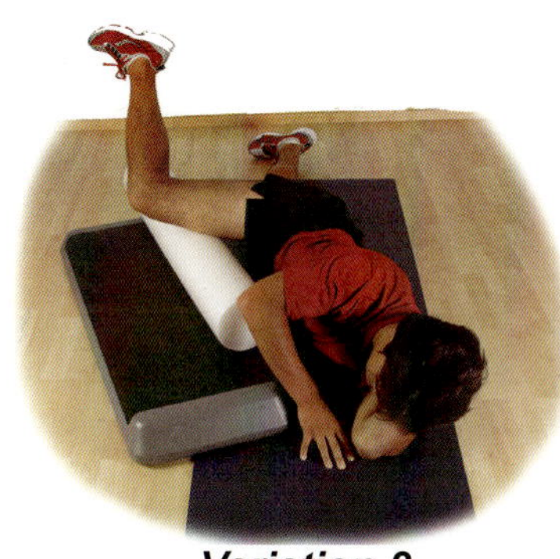

Variation 2

Myofascial Release

Hamstring Release

Purpose: Massages hamstrings.

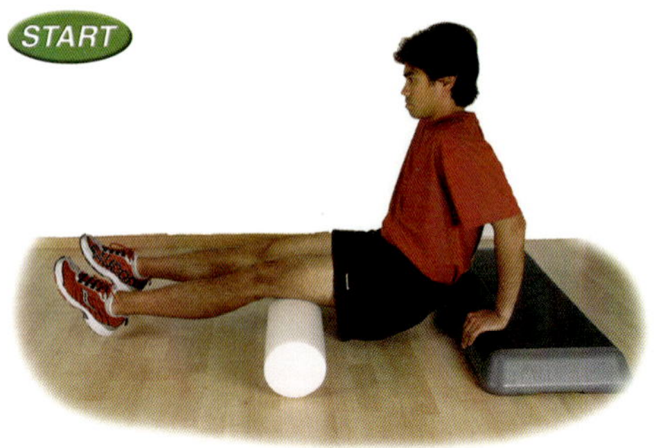

1. Place a full roller on the floor.
2. Sit with your buttocks hanging off the back of the roller.
3. Place your hands behind you on the floor, or on an elevated flat surface, for support.
4. Extend your legs straight in front of you – keep them slightly raised off the floor.
5. Perform the Girdle Grip (pg. 8).
6. Gently roll back and forth, massaging the backs of your thighs, feeling for pain spots.
7. Once you find a tender spot, roll over it firmly until you feel the tension release.
8. Then feel for another pain spot.

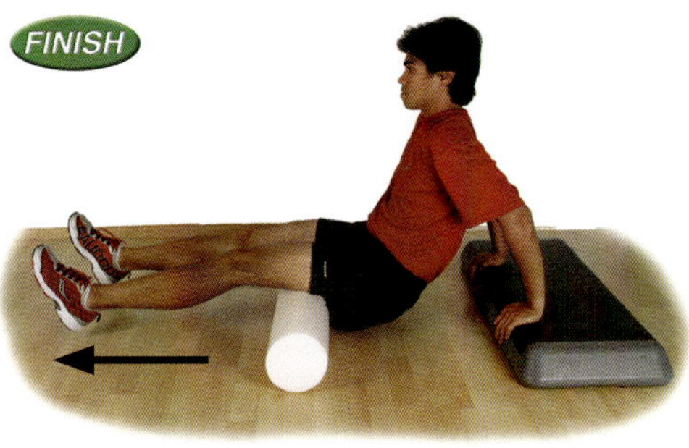

Variations:

1. With your legs still raised, turn your toes inward. Rolling back and forth will now massage the inside hamstrings.
2. Then turn your toes outward to massage the outside hamstrings.

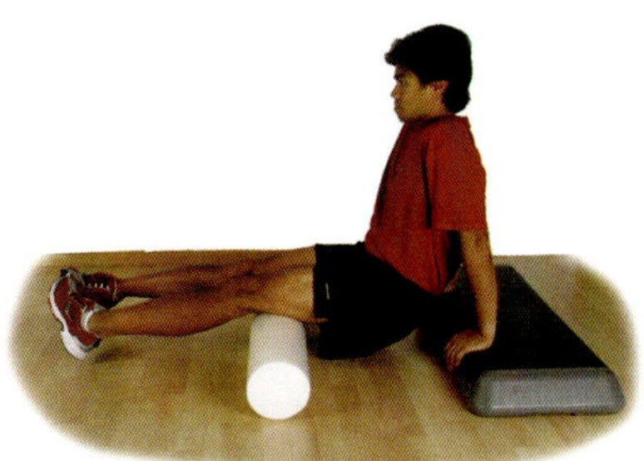

Toes in

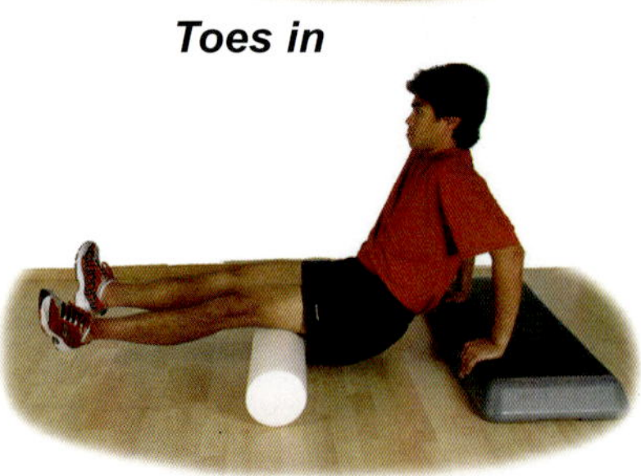

Toes out

Calf Release

Purpose: Massages calves: Toes in = medial head of gastrocnemius, Toes out = lateral head of gastrocnemius.

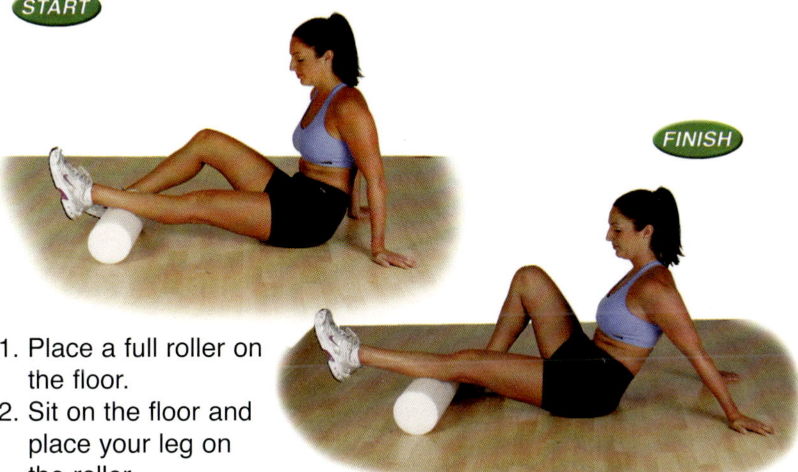

1. Place a full roller on the floor.
2. Sit on the floor and place your leg on the roller.
3. Position the roller against your calf muscle, just above the ankle.
4. Place your hands behind you on the floor for support.
5. Gently roll back and forth, massaging your calf muscle, feeling for pain spots.
6. Once you find a tender spot, roll over it firmly until you feel the tension release.
7. Then feel for another pain spot.
8. Switch sides.

Variations:

1. Turn your toes inward to massage the inside calf.
2. Turn your toes outward to massage the outside calf.

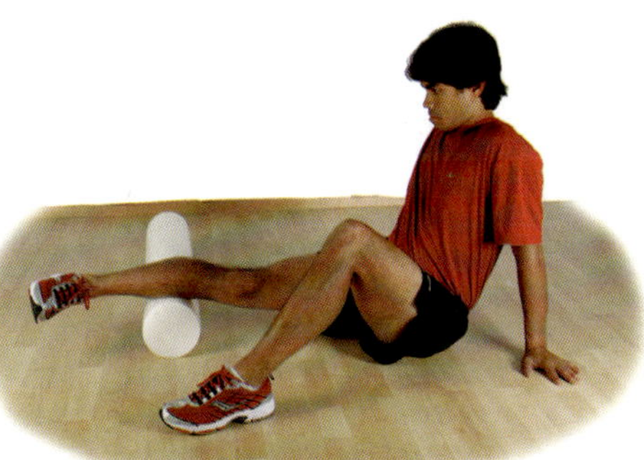

Toes in

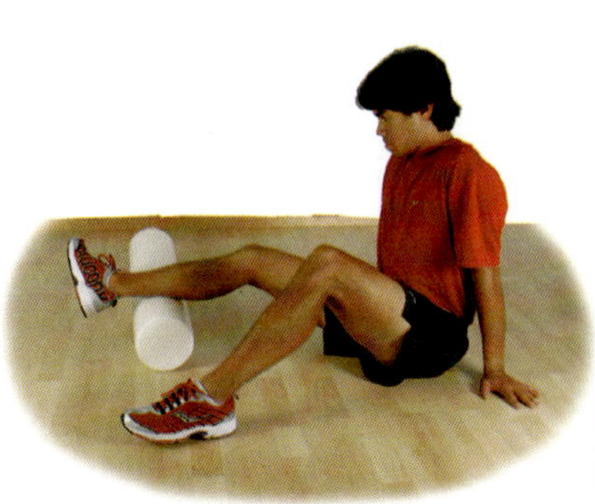

Toes out

Other Products by
Productive Fitness Products Inc.

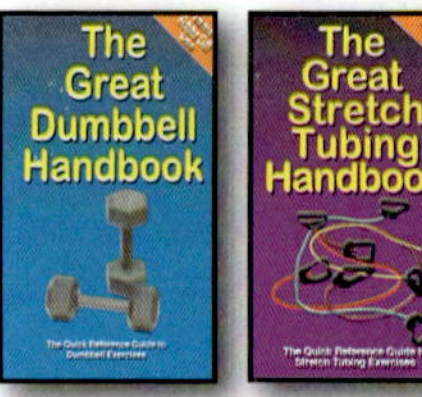

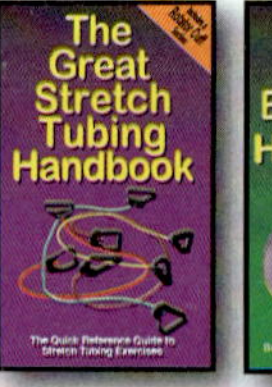

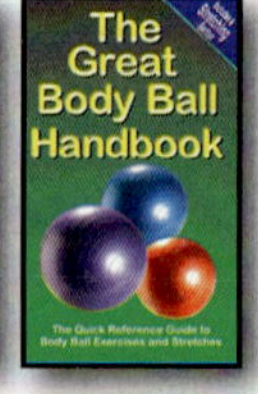

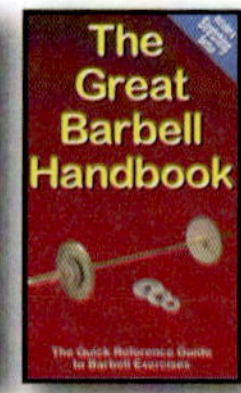

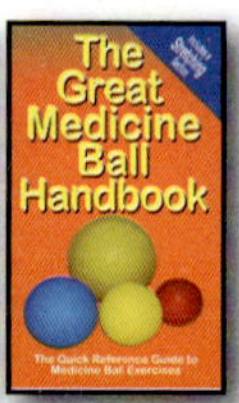

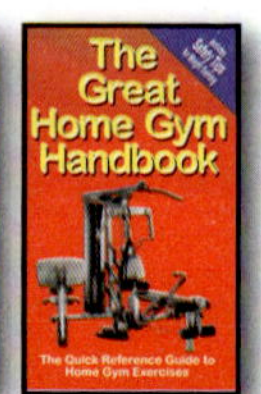

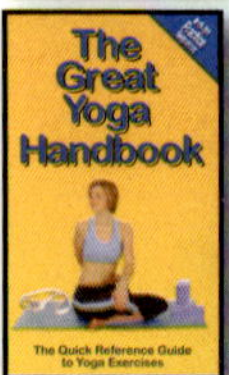

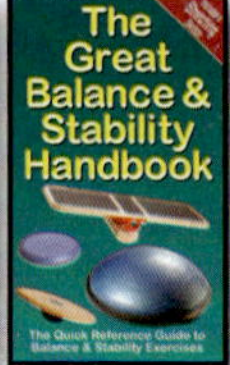

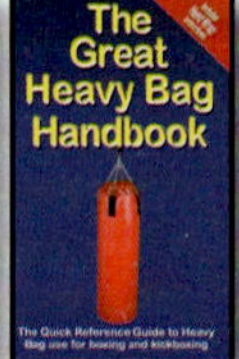

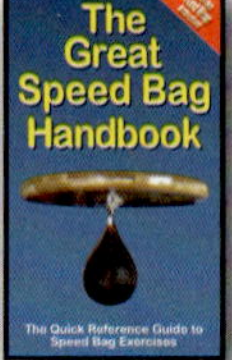

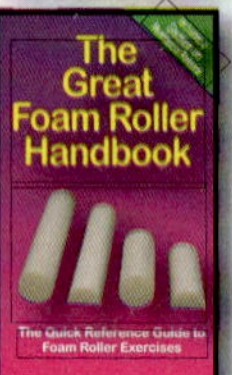

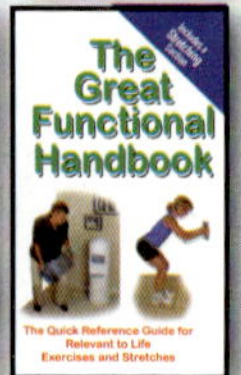

Fitness Poster Series

Full-Color **24" x 36"** Posters sold individually laminated or paper.

Body Ball-Core

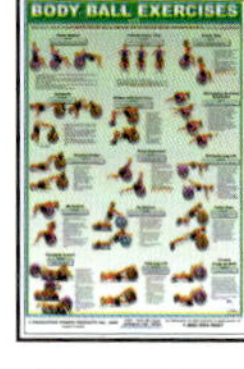

Body Ball Upper/Lower Body

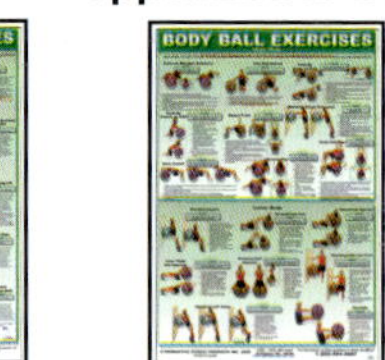
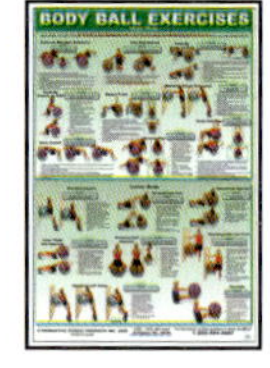

Dumbbell Shoulders/Arms

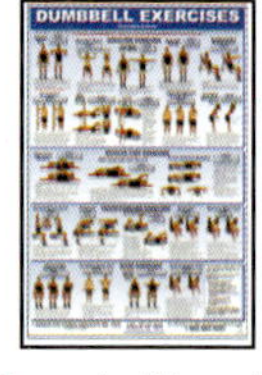

Dumbbell-Lower Body/Core/ Chest/Back

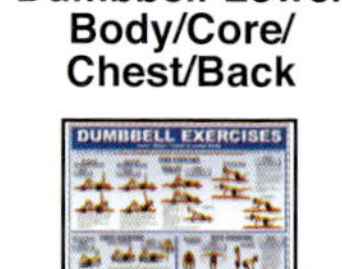

Stretching Upper Body

Stretching Lower Body

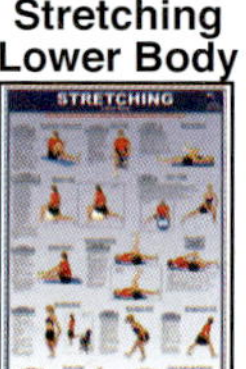

Female Muscle Diagram

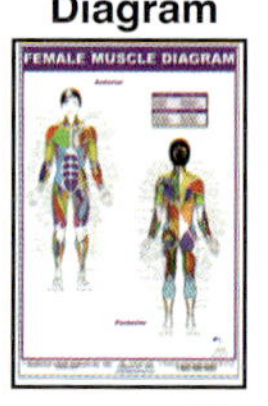

Male Muscle Diagram

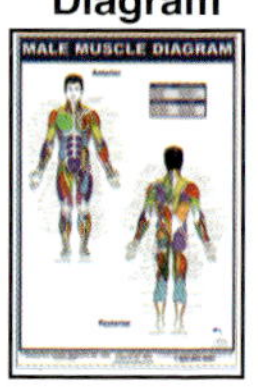

Fitness Heart Rate Chart

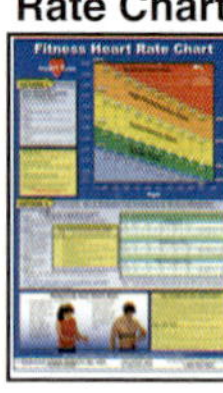

Home Gym Exercises

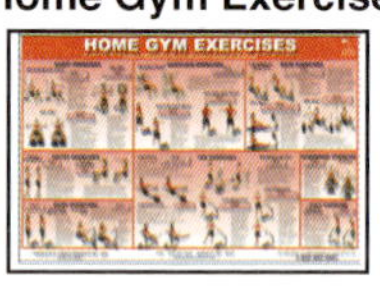

The Ultimate Weight Training Journal

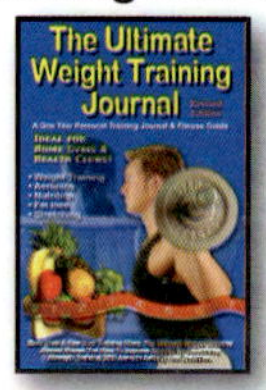

Body Ball Training Poster Pack

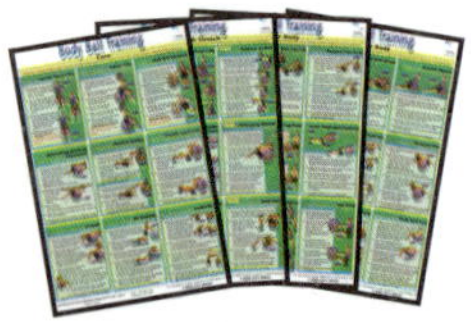

Dumbbell Training Poster Pack

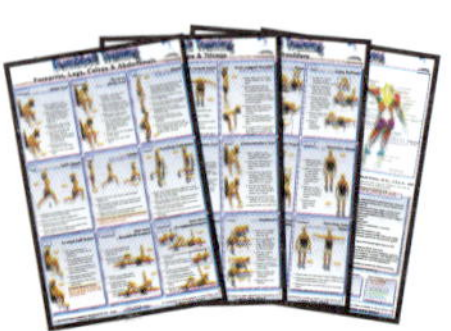

Stretch Tubing Training Poster Pack

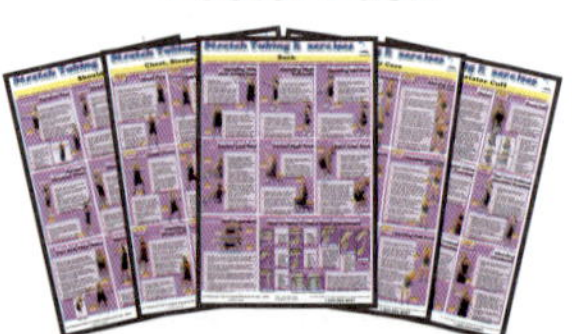